When Hope Never Dies

*One Woman's Remarkable Recovery
from Cancer—and the Natural
Program that Saved Her Life*

Marlene McKenna
with Tom Monte

KENSINGTON BOOKS
http://www.kensingtonbooks.com

The contents of this book reflect the author's philosophy, beliefs, and personal experience. The ideas and suggestions contained in this book are not intended to be a substitute for consultation with your own physician. If medical advice is required, the services of a competent professional should be sought.

KENSINGTON BOOKS are published by

Kensington Publishing Corp.
850 Third Avenue
New York, NY 10022

ISBN 1-57566-509-3

First Printing: February, 2000
10 9 8 7 6 5 4 3 2 1

Printed in the United States of America

When Hope Never Dies

Contents

Introduction

On March 19, 1986, I was diagnosed with malignant mela-noma that had spread throughout my small intestine. Exploratory surgery had revealed that my small intestine had been infiltrated "extensively" by malignant tumors. My surgeon explained to me that there was nothing else conventional medicine could do for me and that my only hope—however slim that was—lay with one or another of the experimental cancer therapies being offered at the National Cancer Institute or at Yale Medical Center. Short of a miracle, I had between six months to a year to live. I was forty years old, married, and the mother of four children.

The diagnosis of cancer was so shocking and terrible that for weeks I felt as if I had lost touch with myself and my surroundings. In a way, I disengaged from my world. I went inward and hid myself from all that I was feeling. My husband, Keven, did his best to support me. We both said all the right words one expects to say in the face of such a crisis: "We'll fight it," we said. "We'll beat this thing. We'll explore all the cutting-edge treatments and get the best therapy possible. Somehow we'll find a way."

Even as I said those words, I felt removed from them—and from my life. I was numb. Whenever I did reconnect with myself and my circumstances, whenever I allowed myself to feel what was really going on inside me, I was immediately overwhelmed with fear and sadness. The toughest times of all came during the little moments with the children—when I saw them go off to school in the morning, or when I tucked my youngest, Mary Kathryn, into bed at night. How could I leave them? How could this happen to me, especially at my age? When I considered my situation and my fate, I was soon overcome by panic. I could only take so much fear before I switched back to automatic pilot, as if my soul detached itself from my body and mind. Once again, I resumed a kind of numb detachment. I went through the day as if only half of me was present.

In hindsight I realized that those symptoms were the outward expression of a life completely out of balance. Essentially, I raced through every day, meeting the demands of my work and family. The central motivations behind most of my actions were my career and financial goals, which took up most of my time and energy. As for my other priorities, my children and my husband came next. If someone had asked me what I did for myself or whether I spent any time with myself, I would have laughed politely and said, "I am with myself all day long. Everything I do is for me, in some way." In other words, I would not even have understood the question, because I didn't know what it meant to be truly in touch with the inner me.

I must admit that I didn't have the slightest understanding of what the word "balance" meant. I cannot remember actually using the word before I got cancer. Later, after I began to truly dedicate myself to recovering my health, I realized that only by living a balanced life could I enjoy some degree of intimacy with myself, that I could actually be aware of my inner world—that I might actually be aware of who I am. Only by having such an awareness could I know my own physical, emotional, and psychological needs, which of course is the first step toward meeting those needs.

In a very real sense, cancer awakened me to the blind rush in which I lived. After the shock of my diagnosis began to wear off and I started to feel again, I turned within, searching for that part of me that would endure beyond death. That inner world, with its gentle, nurturing, and reassuring voice, was the gateway to spiritual life, which was the only thing that stood between me and terror. Not only did it give me hope, but it was my guide to an endless number of practical decisions. Each day, my inner life directed me intuitively, helping me decide what I must do next to strengthen my health and, eventually, overcome my cancer. In an odd sort of paradox, surrendering to the inner world gave me the answers to the outer one. Directed by my inner voice, I sought and found people who helped me out of my fear and confusion. Ultimately, they even helped me find an answer to my disease.

In the pages that follow, I share my journey from sickness to health, from hopelessness to the restoration of my life. More than anything else, I want my readers to know that no one can tell you with absolute certainty what you are capable of accomplishing, even when all the odds seem stacked against you. I was told that there was no hope of recovery from malignant melanoma. Certainly, the doctors who assured me that my fate was sealed were speaking from experience. Yet, I did recover. When I look back, it seems as if I was being led—indeed, I believe I was. But while in the midst of my recovery process, I felt alone and afraid much of the time. What got me through the experience were my faith and a set of daily health practices that gave me the means to help myself and keep me grounded in the here and now. My macrobiotic diet and lifestyle, my meditations, exercise, and daily yoga were the practical activities that I used every day to strengthen my body, mind, and spirit. These are powerful tools and they worked for me.

Faith and action formed the basis of my recovery. They are the yin and yang of what I came to see as true self-empowerment. Faith alone, I came to realize, is ungrounded and impractical. In a very real sense, faith alone is not really faith but desperate fear masquerading as faith. On the other hand, daily health practices without faith is pure futility. What can we accomplish if we do not believe in what we are doing? Faith and action became, for me, the mingling of heaven and earth. In this way, I was being guided; I believed my actions were inspired by a higher power.

Faith and action are also the basis for peace. At some point, I realized that if I survived this ordeal, eventually there would be another one that I would not survive. What mattered to me in the end, therefore, was that I became transformed so that I might better accept what I perceived to be the divine plan for my life. It was my responsibility to do all I could do to get well. There was no escaping that effort, especially since it was that very act that offered me the means to understand and transform my life.

By writing this book, I encourage you to find your own way, to discover what works for you. While you search for healing tools, never lose your practical common sense. Ideally, every healing method should make you feel physically and mentally better; it should have an impact on your disease; and it should grant you greater access to your own inner self. My approach gave me all three gifts, which is why I want to share my experience with you.

Part One

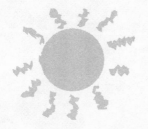

CHAPTER 1

The Wrecking Ball

Spring was coming. The March air was cold and there was a stiff wind that still had to be faced, but the sun was getting stronger and the days just a little longer. There were suggestions, here and there, that nature was about to rebound yet again, despite the awesome power of winter to snuff out all but the faintest embers of life. Spring always brings hope, I thought again, as I stood in my kitchen at the sink and filled a teapot with water. I had to keep focusing on the positive. Somehow I would find a way out of this terrible nightmare.

I would be admitted to Massachusetts General Hospital in Boston the following day to undergo exploratory surgery, but my health had been collapsing in stages.

Three years before, I had been diagnosed with malignant melanoma. After a malignant mole had been removed from my back, I entered a frightening period in which new signs of disease seemed to emerge with shocking regularity. With each new symptom my life seemed driven all the closer to some perilous cliff. For most of that three-year period, my doctors were unable to determine what exactly was wrong with me. None of them wanted to jump to the obvious conclusion: The melanoma had recurred and my symptoms were not as mysterious and inexplicable as they were saying. Finally, in February 1986, the obvious was inescapable. Yes, my doctors finally acknowledged, the cancer probably had returned. I would have to undergo exploratory surgery to confirm or deny everyone's suspicions.

Now, in my kitchen on the day before I was to be admitted to the hospital, I couldn't help but consider my life and the events that had brought me to this terrible precipice.

I was born on May 3, 1946, and raised in Rhode Island. I had a traditional Roman Catholic upbringing, attended Skidmore College in New York, and graduated with a degree in government. After graduation I attended the School of Advanced International Studies in Paris, France, an opportunity that was made possible by my fluency in French. In 1970 I enrolled in a graduate program at the University of Rhode Island and began working on an advanced degree in government, economics, and history. Two years later I met Keven McKenna, also a native of Rhode Island, who was just finishing law school at Georgetown Law in Washington, D.C. In 1973 we married.

We made our home in Providence and began a family. Keven had had two children by a previous marriage and within four years we had added two more. Keven developed his law practice, and while the children were young, I stayed home to raise them.

Keven and I loved government and politics, and these were exciting days for us. He rose within the ranks of the Democratic Party and in 1976 ran for lieutenant governor, only to lose by fewer than eight thousand votes. Two years later he ran for state attorney general and lost, but was later elected to three terms in the state legislature. In 1985 he was elected as a delegate to the 1986 State Constitutional Convention and served as the convention president. Eventually, he was elected by the city council as a municipal court judge of Providence. Meanwhile, he continued his law practice.

I became a stockbroker and financial planner in 1977, dividing my time between family and work. For much of the next nine years, my career steadily rose, consuming more and more of my time, energy, and mental focus. As a consequence of our jobs, Keven and I were continually on the go.

I learned early in my career that being a woman in the world of finance was a distinct disadvantage. In 1978 executives at a prestigious Wall Street firm refused to promote me after promising me a higher position within the firm. I sued the corporation for sex discrimination and won. People said that my suit would effectively banish me from the financial-services industry. They were wrong. I joined a retail brokerage firm, Janney Montgomery-Scott, began doing investment and finance commentary on local radio, and eventually became a weekly commentator for investments and finance on WJAR-TV in Providence.

In fact, within a few years of my suit, I became an associate vice president at Shearson Lehman Hutton. I was proud of my success and took for granted that it entailed living under continuous stress. The needs of my work and family were essentially my puppet strings: they directed me to meet so-and-so for a business meeting, pulled me to satisfy an endless series of deadlines—make sure my children got their homework done, that they were bathed, clothed, and well-fed, that they got to their track meets or basketball games, that the house was tidy.

I actually thought by racing to *this* meeting, or completing my work to meet *that* deadline, I was meeting my needs. Like so many other Americans, I believed that living was "doing." The possibility that I could just *be*—that I could just experience my life without having to accomplish anything—never occurred to me. When I wasn't doing something, I was wasting time, I thought.

One of the clearest manifestations of imbalance in my life—though I didn't realize it at the time—was that I was continually attempting to suppress my own feminine side and promote my more masculine characteristics. The world of finance, especially in the 1970s and '80s, is a man's world and dominated by male-behavior patterns. In order to make it in the world of finance, I fostered the masculine within me, and neglected the feminine in all its manifestations. I constantly initiated new projects; I chased every opportunity that came my way. I worried—some say, I obsessed—about the small details. I was aggressive and ambitious; I disdained rest. I saw little value in receptivity, unless it made a client trust me; in listening to my inner voice, unless it proved to be an accurate hunch in the stock market; in balance, unless we were talking about my checkbook. I was on the fast track to success. But as my career rose, my health steadily declined.

The warning signs had been there for years. My body had been developing tiny tumors that I would discover at odd moments—when going to the bathroom, for example, or while combing my hair before a mirror. My mind would be elsewhere, with my job or children, or on some meaningless chore that had to be attended to shortly, and then my hand or my eye would stumble upon an unusual bump. It was as if another part of my brain had directed my attention there instinctively, and suddenly my entire life would be focused on a tiny growth no bigger than a pea. Flames of fear would rise spontaneously from my stomach and chest and then envelop me. What was this thing? What was happening to me? I would run through a whole litany of fearful possibilities and then I would run to my doctor.

Each time the cyst would be examined and given its proper classification in very specific medical terms. The cysts began appearing in April 1978, when I developed a sebaceous cyst on my sex organs. Over the next five years, they appeared regularly, beginning with a "chalazion" (or cyst) over my right eye, and a "lipoma" (or fatty tumor) on my back; then a subcutaneous nodule on my back, and a keratotic lesion (or hard, raised growth) on my chest; next a pigmented lesion on my right palm, another on my abdomen, and still another on my neck.

These growths suggested nothing to my physicians, save for the fact that some of them needed to be removed. In fact, there was nothing more any doctor could do for me. Physicians had no understanding of why the body might produce cysts, or what might be done about them.

Only my husband and I seemed to discern a dangerous pattern. Clearly, something inside of me was causing the production of these tumors, I believed. All I ever got from my doctors was a name for my latest growth or the recommendation of a surgeon who would remove it. At night Keven and I would sometimes discuss my health and the lack of any fundamental treatment that might stop me from producing these frightening growths. There was no such treatment available, it seemed. At that point we recognized the enormous difference between diagnosis, or the act of naming something, and real treatment. Meanwhile, I felt utterly powerless.

The Other Shoe Drops

And then on August 23, 1983, the foundation of my life started cracking. On that day I told my doctor, Marla Angermeier, that I had noticed a change in a mole on the right upper part of my back. The growth had been bothering me for several months. It had become itchy and recently started to bleed. I was afraid that the mole had become enlarged, too.

On my medical record, Dr. Angermeier noted a "2.5 to 3 cm. geographic shaped plaque, ranging in color from light to dark brown, with a few areas of pink." Dr. Angermeier said that part of the lesion would have to be removed and evaluated as a possible cancer. She then performed what is called a "punch biopsy," meaning that a small piece of the tumor was removed and sent to a lab at a local hospital to be assayed. Two days later, Keven and I were back in Dr. Angermeier's office. As always, she was direct. She informed me that the report had come back from the hospital lab indicating that the tumor was malignant and that there was "a very mild lymphocytic infiltrate," meaning that it had penetrated slightly into the tissues of my back. "You have malignant melanoma," she said.

Those words hit my life like a wrecking ball. A haze came over me. I felt as if I were only semiconscious, as if the impact of her words blew the strength out of me. I surrendered to the haze and let Keven get the details.

He questioned Dr. Angermeier on what it all meant. The illness was life-threatening, she said. It may have spread to other parts of my body, in which case it might eventually pass to my brain or some other vital organ and kill me. The tumor would have to be removed, but a surgeon who specializes in cancer would have to determine whether the lymph nodes in my back, neck, and arm would be taken out, as well. Arrangements would have to be made immediately.

Everything happened quickly now. We consulted four different oncologists who gave us four different opinions on what to do with the tumor. Finally we chose a local surgeon who suggested doing a narrow excision and then having the tumor further evaluated. He did that surgery on September 13, 1983. The resulting pathology report stated that I had Clark's Level III melanoma, meaning that it was malignant and perhaps had spread to other parts of my body.

After I had recovered from the operation, my surgeon wanted to remove the lymph nodes from the site of the tumor—on my back, to my waist. He called it "chasing melanoma," meaning removing the lymph nodes to which the cancer might have spread. I was dubious and decided to consult a dermatologist and surgeon at Boston's Massachusetts General Hospital. The dermatologist was blunt with me. "That approach went out ten years ago," he said. "The cancer might have spread to your brain, liver, or other organs. There's no point in chasing it now." In October 1983 he removed a limited number of nodes around the site of the tumor. Also, punch biopsies were done on tumors on my abdomen and left ear, both of which proved benign.

Based on the evaluation at Massachusetts General Hospital, Dr. Angermeier recommended no more surgery, and I felt as if I had reached an unknown shore where I hoped I would be safe.

To this point, I had received the standard medical treatment. The medical strategy for those with precancerous symptoms is essentially, "Let's wait and see." For a person with cancer such an approach is like sitting on a beach while a storm builds just offshore. For most people with such symptoms it's only a matter of time before the storm rises and engulfs them. Once you are diagnosed, you are subjected to the horrors of treatment. Our society has accepted them, but the individual patient undergoes a series of terrible shocks that are themselves difficult to deal with. Still, having emerged from the surgery, with no more treatment scheduled, I clung to the words of my doctors: "It's possible that we got it all." But in fact I had entered Wonderland, where the events seemed controlled by a power all their own.

When Everything Tumbles Toward Oblivion

Only a few weeks after my surgery I noticed that I had developed a lump on the back of my neck, near the spine. Initially I tried to dismiss it, but to my horror the lump clearly began to grow. On February 8, 1984, I went to Dr.

Angermeier and reported the growth. A "subcutaneous nod-ule," she called it. It was small, moved freely, and appeared almost innocent. We'd watch it, she told me.

After the discovery of the subcutaneous nodule, I found another lipoma, which was biopsied by Dr. Angermeier. A few melanoma cells were discovered beneath the fatty tissue. Initially Dr. Angermeier and a surgeon at my HMO recom-mended that all the lymph nodes in my neck be removed, but Dr. A. Benedict Cosimi, a surgeon at Massachusetts General, recommended a limited removal of lymph nodes from the right side of the neck, which he did in July 1984. He did not find any cancer in the lymph nodes. I would therefore not need chemotherapy, he said. No further treatment was rec-ommended.

The fact that I was not getting any further treatment did not in any way allay my fears, however. On the contrary, I had good reason to be afraid of what was happening to me be-cause other frightening signs began to emerge: I developed a lesion on my chest—a keratotic papule, it was called. I also developed another lesion on my chest that Dr. Angermeier referred to as a "flesh-colored papule with some very dark reticulated pigmentation in it." In March 1985 two papules emerged—one on each of my eyebrows. Dr. Angermeier of-fered that I could have "elective surgery" to remove the growths. Other growths emerged with frightening regularity.

With each new symptom, I would see yet another specialist and undergo another round of tests, none of which proved par-ticularly revealing. This frustrated and terrified me because it was obvious that my physicians had no answers for me.

In August I developed acute abdominal pain after horse-back riding one afternoon. I thought the jostling of my stom-ach may have brought it on. In fact, I had been having chronic, low-grade intestinal problems for the previous eleven years, but after horseback riding, the intestinal trou-ble became acute.

In September my HMO turned me over to yet another

physician, this time a specialist in gastrointestinal disorders, whom I will call Dr. Jones. Dr. Jones did no tests on me, but informed me that I had spastic colon. "What is spastic colon?" I asked. The muscles in my intestines were acting up, I was informed. He prescribed Donnatol, a drug designed to relieve intestinal distress.

My problems persisted, however. Soon I was back at Dr. Jones's office, complaining of more intestinal pain. I had also lost ten pounds. I am five feet seven inches tall and thin. The loss of ten pounds frightened me.

At our second meeting he said that the weight loss was due to lactose intolerance, or indigestion caused by my inability to digest the sugar in milk, called lactose. He told me that I should eliminate dairy products from my diet, and placed me on several dietary supplements: daily calcium, vitamins with iron, and 1,000 milligrams of vitamin C. Dr. Jones also noted my history of "metastatic melanoma," but observed in my medical record that my problems were "unlikely to be caused by any significant pathologic process. . . . No evidence of any metastatic disease."

Dr. Jones went further. He attributed my intestinal pain and weight loss to my lifestyle. He explained that I was trying to do too much by trying to balance career and family, and that I was being little more than a hyperactive yuppie.

In the end the condescension with which I was treated by doctors was insulting, to be sure, but more than anything it frightened me. Intuitively I knew there was more wrong with me than stress and a "spastic colon."

Much to my surprise, the elimination of dairy food did alleviate my digestive problems somewhat, but only for a short while. In December the intestinal pain was back. I was vomiting now. Dr. Jones said it was the flu.

My intestinal pain, indigestion, and nausea only got worse. My HMO directed me to another physician, this one a woman who assured me in the most condescending tone possible that nothing was wrong with me.

"Could it be an ulcer?" I asked. "I had ulcers in college."

"No," she said with a polite, dismissive smile that suggested how silly I was being for worrying my little head over medical issues.

"Then why do I have so much pain and these digestive problems?" I asked.

She didn't know, she said. She put a note in my medical record that reflected the tone of our discussion. "The patient is wondering whether this is ulcer disease," the doctor wrote. "I tried to explain to her that she really did not seem to be having any of the signs or symptoms of ulcer but she seemed fairly insistent on that."

She gave me nothing to treat my distress. But she did note in my record that I had "good bowel sounds."

Keven argued with my physicians that they were treating me as if I were a hypochondriac. "You're saying that there really is nothing wrong with Marlene," Keven told Dr. Jones, "and that if she just settles down and relaxes, she'll be okay. But we believe that there is some kind of organic disease here and we're concerned, to say the least." We were both assured that all the examinations and tests had revealed nothing untoward about my condition and that in time my body would right itself.

Meanwhile, my intestinal problems not only continued but grew worse. By February 1986 I was back in the office of my internist, complaining of abdominal pain, vomiting, and dizzy spells. My weight had now fallen to 105 pounds. The doctor ordered that I be admitted to Miriam Hospital in Providence for a full battery of tests. I noted a bit ruefully that she recorded my "history of bleeding ulcers" in my medical report.

At Miriam it was discovered that I had internal bleeding, for which I required four units of blood. I spent four days in the hospital, where I was confronted with a new round of doctors and an array of medical tests, including an upper G.I. series using barium meal. The tests showed that I had a small hiatal hernia and fluid in the abdominal cavity, and that the small intestine had dilated loops, which suggested an obstruction within the organ. However, doctors noted that the barium flowed through my intestines easily. No one knew what the obstruction might be.

Unfortunately, when the barium test was concluded, no one bothered to remove the barium from my intestinal tract. Barium meal is made of metallic particles that prevent X rays from passing through the tissue, and thus allow physicians to see the shape of the intestine.

After I left the hospital, the barium began to harden. Eventually it felt like concrete in my gut. My stomach swelled and I looked four-months pregnant. Meanwhile, the pain became almost unbearable. As I writhed in pain, the thought occurred to me that maybe the doctors should have given me something to eliminate the barium from my intestines. I called the head nurse at the hospital and asked if the barium should have been removed.

"Yes," she said. "Wasn't it?"

"No, it wasn't," I screamed.

The responsibility for ordering the barium removed from my system was my doctor's. Since he did not order it, nobody did it. It was that simple. Desperate for relief, I performed the enemas myself. For the next two weeks, my intestines felt like they were carrying around a lot of loose cement. The pain intensified and I was ordered back to Miriam Hospital for another round of tests and possible treatment.

Keven was beside himself with frustration. "You guys are not being good enough detectives," he screamed at the doctor. "Something is wrong with my wife and you're not getting to the bottom of it."

Keven finally let out his frustrations on one doctor, saying, "What is this, an assembly line? The Henry Ford approach to health care? We have specialists for Marlene's skin cancer, specialists for her intestines, specialists for her gynecological concerns, and we've got surgeons thrown into the mix. I don't think anyone is really backing up and looking at the whole person. Each of you is looking at Marlene and her tests from your own narrow specialty. Each of you wants more and more tests, and none of those tests prove conclusive."

My condition rapidly worsened from this point onward. My hematocrit test, which measures the percentage of red blood cells packed into a volume of blood, was at twenty percent, well below the thirty-eight to forty-six percent that is normal for an adult woman. By late February my doctors finally began to acknowledge the obvious: In all likelihood, my cancer had spread to my small intestine.

On March 19, 1986, I was admitted to Massachusetts General Hospital, where exploratory surgery discovered multiple cancerous lesions in my small intestine. Dr. Cosimi, my surgeon, reported his findings: "Not unexpectedly, rather extensive metastatic disease to the small bowel was encountered. There were two segments of small bowel containing a total of five separate lesions that required resection . . . there was considerable lymphadenopathy throughout the mesentery of the small bowel," meaning swelling of the lymph nodes within my small intestine and in the tissues just outside of it.

Dr. Cosimi removed twenty-two inches of my small intestine, taking the obvious cancerous tumors that existed in that part of the organ. He left no doubt that other cancerous lesions still existed within me. "Undoubtedly, she has other positive nodes in the mesentery and perhaps other occult lesions in the bowel, as well," he later reported. "It would be appropriate, therefore, to proceed with some form of adjuvant therapy at this time. We recommend combined chemo/immunotherapy. . . . Certainly reasonable for her to look into the interferon program at Yale."

When I had been moved from the recovery room to my hospital room, Keven sat holding the ends of my fingers—one of the few parts of me, it seemed, that was not punctured by intravenous needles or attached to a tube.

"The kids want to come up and see you," he said.

"Can we wait until after they take out all this stuff?" I asked. "They're just going to frighten the children."

"Okay," he said. He patted my hand and smiled.

A few days later, Damian, my eleven-year-old, and Mary Kathryn, who was eight, came running into my hospital room and embraced me while I lay in bed. They had big smiles on their faces. How little they know, I thought to myself. And then I thought, That's good.

They wanted to walk around the hospital with me. I wanted to walk, too, but the nurse insisted I ride in a wheelchair. Once I was in the chair, the two children started fighting over who was going to push me first. When we had negotiated an amicable arrangement, all four of us started down the hallway.

The corridor was busy. Family members pushed patients through the hallway or helped them on walkers. Hospital personnel hurried up and down the hall. Now and then, a gurney passed us by. Suddenly, we heard exotic music emanating from one of the rooms farther down the hall. As we got closer, I recognized the sultry twanging sound of a dulcimer and the clanging of finger cymbals. It was the music of the Middle East. The dulcimer was clearly a recording, but the cymbals sounded as if they were being played by someone in the room itself. We approached the room with a mixture of curiosity and caution, apprehensive that we might intrude on someone.

We reached the door and peeked inside. Whatever I expected, it wasn't this: a belly dancer performing for a man lying in the hospital bed. She was dressed in the belly dancer's traditional costume. Her maroon top, which exposed her midriff, was trimmed in gold, as were her yellow silken pants. As she danced, she snapped tiny finger cymbals. The man in the hospital bed never took his eyes off her, nor did she look at any of us. Meanwhile, the music swirled about the room, like the dancer herself, and momentarily transported all of us to faraway lands.

The children were awestruck. I was amused but also a little embarrassed for them. Keven and I looked at each other and smiled. "Okay," he whispered after a moment. "Let's go."

Once free of the spell created by the music and the scene, the children broke out in laughter. Suddenly Damian was pushing me a little faster down the hallway and Mary Kathryn was imitating, as best she could, the belly dancer's movements.

"You never know what you're going to see in life, kids," I said.

When I was discharged from the hospital, I was told that I had between six months and a year to live. Based on the existing research and the current assessments of my condition, I could not expect to live beyond one year. I would probably die sooner. The way I would die, I was told, was that the cancer would migrate to one of my vital organs, such as the brain, lungs, or liver, destroy the organ and eventually kill me.

Anyone looking at me would have questioned whether I would last a month. I was emaciated, my weight had fallen to the nineties. I was pale, and my stomach was distended.

Once I was out of the hospital, I took a leave of absence from my job to devote myself to whatever cancer therapy I would undergo. Keven and I made plans to search out all the medically authorized "experimental" cancer treatments. We were both panic-stricken and desperate. As far as my doctors were concerned, I didn't have a prayer, but that was all I could think to do.

CHAPTER 2

Hoping for a Medical Miracle

It's remarkable how that tiny spark of hope stays alive inside of you, even when all the evidence tells you that your situation is hopeless. Perhaps hope is implicit in the spark of life. As I sank to the very bottom of life's trough, I came to realize that as long as there was some life within me, there was still hope—at least a tiny bit of it. But that was precisely my problem. There wasn't much life left in me. At ninety pounds I was as bony and frail as a prisoner of war. I had so little vitality that I felt my life force had all but dried up. Whenever I looked into the mirror, my heart sank. Puffy dark circles surrounded my large brown eyes and sagged with resignation; my mouth was drawn down, exhausted; my skin, gray and lifeless in the main, was punctuated here and there by dark brown patches. Death was as close as the image in the mirror. Or as close as an examination of my own body.

My back and chest were marked by numerous tiny tumors. Dark mounds of tissue, like hardened scabs, or hard pimple-like eruptions, had been emerging from my skin for years. They continued to emerge after I had the surgery. For reasons I could not understand, I continued to produce tumors on the upper part of my body. They terrified me, in part because they served as a periodic reminder of the terrible cancer inside of me. These little bumps and eruptions seemed to me to be cancer's way of telling me that it was still very much alive inside of me and growing all the time.

Still, that little spark of hope endured, driving me forward to the great institutions for cancer research—Boston's New England Medical Center and the Dana Farber Cancer Institute, and the Yale Medical Center of New Haven, Connecticut. Entering these places, I hoped that some wise and even fatherly scientist would give me the answer that would save my life. Though I would have been loath to admit it, I was looking for just a little comfort from these people, some rational reason to hope that I might survive. Despite all my experience with doctors and medicine, I still held out hope that some cutting-edge therapy would save me.

Keven had already done considerable research in the library on the three programs that we were now about to investigate. He had also made telephone calls to talk to researchers. There were three different experimental treatments that were being used on malignant melanoma: the New England Medical Center, where researchers were experimenting with the use of interleukin II, an antibody that scientists hoped would kill the cancer; the Dana Farber Cancer Institute, where researchers were studying the use of bone marrow transplant in the treatment of melanoma; and the Yale Medical Center, where scientists were studying interferon as a potential cancer treatment.

Keven and I went first to the New England Medical Center, where a scientist told us that I was not eligible for the interleukin II program, due to the fact that I did not have an exposed tumor, which is the only kind of tumors they were working on at the time. My skin tumors had been removed. The active cancer that was in me now was in my intestinal tract, and God knew where else. Thus, I was quickly dismissed as a candidate for that program.

Our next appointment was at the Yale Medical Center in New Haven, where scientists were studying the effects of interferon on cancer, including malignant melanoma.

In a sterile little office that seemed to belong to no one in particular, we met a physician-scientist who appeared to be in his early forties. He had blond hair and wore glasses and a white lab coat. He was very thin and oddly distant, as if he were talking to us from very far away. Occasionally, when he turned his head, the fluorescent lights above his desk caused a glare to come off his glasses, preventing me from looking into his eyes. The effect was to increase the distance that already existed between us.

I was so weakened at this point that I did not have the strength to engage the physician. Instead, I asked Keven to do most of the talking.

The doctor began by offering what sounded to me like indirect hope that interferon might be an answer for me. "We are hopeful that this therapy might eventually be effective in the treatment of your type of cancer."

Keven cut to the quick. "What are the chances that Marlene might be cured by this treatment, Doctor?"

"At this point, the chances are small," he said. "That doesn't mean that your wife might not benefit. We are studying this method continuously and making adjustments to increase its potential efficacy."

"How small?" Keven asked.

"Right now, I'd say less than one-in-ten."

"What are the side effects?"

As it turned out, the potential side effects were numerous and sometimes severe, including gastrointestinal disorders, immune reactions, joint pain, and death. One doesn't simply die from these treatments, however. One suffers considerably before dying. I must admit that the side effects of all cancer therapy frightened me. I had already been through so much with doctors. Weakened now and at the very edge of my own existence, I didn't think I could take much more pain or discomfort. I wanted my body to heal; exposing it to more pain did not seem like a comforting thought, nor a very practical one.

After listening to all the side effects and the appalling lack of success, I knew that I was better off taking my chances with the cancer. Besides, as I had told Keven, if death was inevitable, I wanted to limit the suffering as much as I could. Keven asked the doctor a few more questions, ending with whether there was anything the doctor knew about that might be an effective treatment for melanoma.

"Aside from what we are doing," he answered, "I know of nothing that offers any hope."

I had to bite back the words that were on the tip of my tongue: Your program doesn't offer any hope, either. We all shook hands and parted. As Keven and I left the office, I noticed that the doctor's demeanor had not changed one bit. A polite smile remained on his lips. I had the feeling that our presence—and the desperation of my cause—had not made the slightest impression on him.

Next we went to Dana Farber to discuss the possibility of my getting into the bone marrow transplant program, or what the scientists there were calling the stamp program. We knew already that this treatment was being used as a possible therapy for malignant melanoma; what we didn't know were the study's results to this point. Perhaps recent results had been more promising; perhaps there had even been a few cures. This was our thinking when we arrived.

In a small conference room at the hospital, we met a doctor in his mid-fifties, overweight, and balding. In the most euphemistic and indirect language possible, he explained to us that the results of his research—the use of bone marrow transplant on patients with malignant melanoma—had not been promising to this point. "We will continue to study the possible use of this therapy," he said. "You are eligible for the program and we could enroll you within a few weeks." He gave me the dates when the next round of treatments would occur. He then made some general comments that, I presumed, were intended to hold out some hope that the treatment might work in me.

"Have you seen anyone who has been cured from this treatment?" Keven asked.

"So far, we have not had much success with the treatment. We are still hopeful, however."

"Well, can you tell us anything?" Keven asked. "We have found that many of these experimental treatments have severe side effects, and some can be lethal."

"Only one-in-ten people have died from the treatment," the doctor responded.

Shocked, Keven looked at the man. "If that's your criteria for success, Doctor, we're in deep trouble," he said. His words fell on the room like a mortar shell. No one knew what to say after Keven's salvo had landed. The silence was suddenly loud.

"What are the side effects to the treatment?" I asked.

The doctor answered at length. "Most of the side effects involve the gastrointestinal tract: diarrhea, nausea, vomiting. About a third of patients experience skin rashes. There is a very real threat of serious infection. Bone marrow transplant requires that we suppress the patient's immune system to keep it from rejecting the donor bone marrow. To do this, we use immunosuppressive agents to dampen the immune response, but there can be complications. The weakened immune system can leave her open to infections from opportunistic organisms. On the other hand, when the immunosuppressive drugs fail, death can occur."

The doctor then went on to say that everything possible would be done to minimize the side effects and keep me comfortable.

Was he making his pitch for bodies? I wondered.

"Nothing you have said makes me think that this is an effective therapy," Keven finally said. "I haven't heard anything that would suggest that it's even worth the gamble." The doctor stared back at Keven with a blank look on his face.

"We believe that at some point this may be a viable treatment for some cancers," he said. "We don't know enough yet." With that last sentence, he looked quickly at me, as if measuring me for a hospital gown, and then turned his gaze away.

Keven turned to me and then to the doctor and said, "Thank you for your time." We all got up from the table, shook hands, and parted. As with his colleague at Yale Medical Center, this doctor's expression never changed. Even now, after we had rejected the treatment, his face remained emotionless.

The world of cancer research, it seemed to me, was extremely hard and cold. It was as though the scientists had walled themselves off from the people who came to them, people who were full of emotion and need. In order to do their work, these researchers needed human volunteers. But the truth was, they were not curing cancer. On the contrary, in many cases they were inflicting considerable pain and suffering. They, however, had steeled themselves against that reality. They had erected a wall between themselves and their "subjects." I realized that that wall existed to keep them from feeling and suffering the consequences of their own work. It kept them from having to look into the eyes of people like me who were desperate for any sign of hope. We would pay anything for the opportunity—however slim it might be—to go on living. Talk about easy marks! I was now part of a group of people who might be the most desperate on earth. A raised eyebrow at the right moment, a single positive word wedged in among a lot of negatives—these things would be grasped at and held on to like life itself. Only these men knew exactly how little hope they had to offer. They kept their cards close to their chests. They had their own ambitions, which, in order to be fulfilled, required that they shut the door of their hearts and lure people like me into their worlds.

After visiting all three cancer centers, I called Dr. Cosimi, my surgeon at Mass General, and told him that I would not be undergoing any one of the three experimental treatments that had been proposed. I asked if he knew of any other possible treatments for malignant melanoma.

"You might qualify for chemotherapy, Marlene," Dr. Cosimi said, "but I cannot promise you that you will live any longer with chemotherapy than without it."

Dr. Cosimi and Dr. Angermeier were the two physicians I trusted the most. I knew what he was saying: I was beyond hope of getting any further treatment from medicine that might do me any good.

No Stranger to Premature Death

For reasons that I still do not fully understand, I never asked questions like "Why me, Lord?" or even pitied myself particularly. Perhaps it was because I had always been a survivor. I was trained to put my deepest feelings into a little box, hide them away—even from myself—and then do whatever needed to be done. That's how I got through life, really. If, before I got cancer, someone had asked me if I enjoyed my life, I probably would have said yes, but only because I would have answered without looking deeply into my own heart. The truth was, I never knew what I felt at any given moment of my life. One of the ways I got through life was by avoiding my feelings. I did whatever my schedule demanded I do. I dealt with whatever problem was shouting the loudest at any given moment. I didn't think there was any other way to live.

I dealt with my cancer in much the same way. This disease is what is in front of me now, I told myself. Essentially, my cancer provided another series of things that had to be done.

Instead of running around in the world of finance, I now ran around in the world of medicine. I visited doctors, got examined, and talked to researchers about possible treatment alternatives. The feeling I experienced more than any other was fear. Apart from that, I was aware of very little else. Fear and the ability to wall myself off from my inner emotional state, especially my sadness, was one of the learned behaviors of my childhood.

My father, Albert Peter Marcello, was a big, warm Italian. He was the kind of man who loved to slap people on the back and hug his wife, children, and friends. He used to take me fishing and tell me stories about the fish. He and his brother founded and ran a very successful company that manufactured costume jewelry. By the time I was entering grade school, he had two hundred employees—his was one of the largest jewelry-manufacturing companies in Rhode Island. By most standards, we were a very well-off family. Growing up, I went to the best schools and never wanted for anything.

I was the middle child, between two brothers. Vincent was four years older than I, and Albert, six years younger. Our family went to church every Sunday and I received the standard childhood sacraments of the church, namely Holy Communion and confirmation. One of the most enduring lessons to emerge from my religious training was to pray to St. Jude, the patron saint of lost causes. St. Jude took on all the difficult jobs, our priests told us. For some reason, that little bit of information stuck with me and, many years later, would be an essential part of my faith.

When I was eleven, my father died suddenly of a heart attack. I was devastated. My father was a giant in my eyes. He kept the family protected from the dangers of the outside world. Suddenly the protector was gone.

I reacted to the loss by going into shock. I was virtually comatose. My soul retreated from life itself, leaving my body as a hollow shell to face the world. At my father's funeral, I floated through the proceedings as if I were a ghost. While people cried openly, I stood near his grave and barely reacted. One woman said to another, "Look at Marlene, she isn't even crying at her father's funeral. What's wrong with her?" The words made me feel exposed and wounded. Was I behaving badly? Did I do something wrong? What was expected of me? I didn't know.

I didn't realize it then, but I was in shock. The death of my father while I was still very young had left me traumatized. I did my best to stand up every day and go through the motions of living, but that was all I did. I was numb to both the outer world and my inner state. I couldn't share my feelings, in part because I couldn't reach them myself. But at night, in the privacy of my own bedroom, I cried myself to sleep for weeks. Why did he leave me? Why did God take him? I didn't understand any of it. All I knew was that our family—my mother, brothers, and I—was alone now. And from then on, I lived as if tragedy might strike again at any moment.

My mother, Katherine, was every bit as traumatized as I. And as if her loss were not enough, another crisis immediately ensued. Once my father was dead, his brother attempted to gain control of the business by reducing the value of my mother's share of the company. My mother's only recourse was to go to court, which precipitated a legal battle that lasted seven years. The eventual outcome was a settlement that was meager in comparison to my father's share of the business.

The fragility of our circumstances—and life itself—was seared on her soul. Could she provide for us? How? Would our family fall from the comfortable heights my father kept us in to the depths of poverty?

The stress was terrible. How she managed it, I have no idea. She went back to school to study bookkeeping and got a job. With that, she kept a roof over our heads, food on the table, and clothes on our backs. She even kept all three of us in private schools. Somehow she soldiered on. But not without enormous cost. Her three children witnessed her struggle and naturally felt enormous sympathy for her.

Yet, she did everything she could to maintain a normal life for us and even wanted to please us as much as she could. We lived in the Elmhurst section of Providence, where you could walk to parks and shops. Sometimes I would tag along as my mother ran errands in our neighborhood and when she was finished she would treat me to an ice cream soda, a milk shake, or a coffee frappe at McCarthy's Drugstore. Mr. McCarthy was a friendly and jovial man who always enjoyed chatting with his customers. After he presented me with some ice cream treat, he would love to ask how I liked it. It seemed to give him a vicarious pleasure. Perhaps he could no longer eat ice cream himself, but got tremendous pleasure watching others enjoy it, especially children. During those occasions, there was such a subtle intimacy between my mother and me. She was also enjoying the fact that I took such pleasure in Mr. McCarthy's treat. Through her eyes or her soft, little smile, she communicated how much she loved me.

Despite her attempts at being brave and strong, we saw her vulnerability and wanted desperately to help her in any way we could. One way we helped her was by being brave ourselves, by not letting on too much about our fears, and by doing whatever we could to assist her with the housework, the laundry, and preparing meals. In time, all three of us developed an overwhelming need to protect our mother, just as she attempted to protect us. Even to this day, it is hard for any one of us to ever say a negative word about her. It was as if the desperation of our circumstances bound us all in a single pact: Protect your mother, because she is all you have.

But in the process I lost my own sense of self. As I tried to protect my mother, I got extremely used to putting my own feelings last. Eventually I lost any sense of my feelings entirely. Only after I got cancer and started to slow down did I realize that I never learned how to provide for my own needs, to nurture myself.

Where Love and Fear Collide

All mothers and daughters have complicated relationships, to say the least, and my relationship with my own mother was no different. At bottom, we have always loved and wanted the best for each other. Unfortunately, that was where the simplicity between us ended—and where the complications began. Love makes all of us vulnerable because we so desperately want to protect the people we love. Nothing triggered my mother's sense of vulnerability more than her three children.

Survival was the paramount issue and everything, it seemed, threatened that survival. Fear, as I would later learn in my own life, causes people to do all they can to control situations and other people. My mother loved us dearly. We were all she had left in the world. And she was not going to stand by and allow the unpredictability of life to destroy us.

Thus, driven by love and fear, my mother attempted to control our lives, very often with disastrous consequences. My mother's reaction to life's unknowns, especially those that affected her children, was to manage our lives as best she could. Perhaps because I was the daughter, and seemingly the most vulnerable child, her concerns were strongest for me. It seemed every aspect of my developing womanhood was scrutinized by my mother. She tried to determine how I should dress, whom I could and could not date, and even how I should think regarding boys. Boys were regarded with universal suspicion. Somehow it was communicated to me that boys were vaguely dangerous, though I didn't understand why. All I really knew was that entering womanhood was fraught with fears and vague negative beliefs.

My mother's desire to protect us and even control our lives

persisted for many years. She still intervened in our marriages, especially my own.

Still, given our family's history, I could not blame her overly. Her primary fault was that she was unable to let go. Like a mother bird who is unable to let her chicks leave the nest, my mother refused to let her own children fly away. This was the basis for our conflicts, such as they were. It was also her legacy to me, one that I eventually realized I would have to transcend.

This was the soil on which I was raised and on which my consciousness developed. The loss of my father and the ensuing court battle forged the belief in me that, for the rest of my life, I would have to take care of myself materially. I must become independent and financially secure, I told myself. My father's death made the world seem infinitely more harsh and dangerous. Now I would have to be the strong one. I couldn't let others have a hold on my resources or my direction in life. There was no room for vulnerability.

Becoming ill seemed to call up all of these old feelings of weakness, exposure to danger, and vulnerability. And as before, it wasn't just me who was exposed, but those I loved the most.

But in a very real sense, the death of my father brought about the loss of my mother. The burdens that fell to her were too heavy. She was now a single parent, responsible for our upbringing and our survival. Suddenly there wasn't time to be concerned about the gentle and tender side of my being, the part of me that needed mothering. She had too much on her plate for worrying about that.

It was not lost on me that just as my mother had been preoccupied by her children, I was now overwhelmed by the same feeling. When my life was threatened, I needed to be close to my children in order to protect them and make sure they would be all right. I took full advantage of my leave of absence from work, taking them as often as I could on day trips to Boston or Newport, or to one of the Rhode Island beaches.

Keven and I had decided that we were not going to tell the children very much about my condition because it would only burden them excessively. Looking back, I do not believe that was a correct decision, though it seemed wise at the time. It was true that the knowledge that their mother was dying would have been a terrible weight for them to carry. But on the other hand, my refusal to tell my children just how bad my condition was served as a wall between us.

Our four children, of course, were of very different ages. In 1986, Sean was twenty; Christopher, seventeen; Damian, eleven, and Mary Kathryn, eight. We had, in effect, two different families within one. The two older boys were adults, for all practical purposes. They knew that I was gravely ill, but they didn't know just how perilous my situation was. They did not know I was dying. Their ignorance of my condition was supported by the fact that they had their own lives and were preoccupied with all that they were doing. Sean was in college and Christopher in high school. Both were very caught up with their schoolwork, their social connections, and the many demands in their lives. Damian and Mary Kathryn, both still in grammar school, had an array of extracurricular activities, as well.

Unlike Sean and Christopher, however, Damian and Mary Kathryn were still young children, who very much needed a mother. They knew nothing of my condition. I wanted to preserve their innocence, but I realized that it kept us from a deeper intimacy that I longed for. Part of me wanted to hold them and hug them and tell them everything—that the weeks or months ahead would be our last together. Let's make them special, I wanted to say. But another part of me wanted to hold back, to protect them. As their mother, I wanted to do everything I could to spare them the pain.

The conflict left me feeling as if my heart had been run

through with a sword. I would try as hard as I could to hold back the tears. Sometimes I failed. Whenever I found myself about to cry, I would usually leave the room before it was noticed, but when one of the four did see me with tears in my eyes and asked what was wrong, I said that it was nothing—just some sad thoughts I was having about a friend, but these would pass. Then I would distract myself, or simply become numb.

Sometimes I would take Damian and Mary Kathryn to the beach and watch them play in the sand. Their perfect little bodies seemed so delicate against the endless ocean that rose and fell in front of them. I knew all too well life's unpredictability, its power and harshness. As if in little boats, we make our way across the ocean of life, never knowing what storms lie ahead, or what the outcome will be. These two children seemed much too small and vulnerable to be set out on that ocean. But of the two, Mary Kathryn worried me more, perhaps because I saw myself in her as a little girl who was about to lose a parent; perhaps because I knew all too intimately the need a little girl has for the love and protection of *both* her parents; and perhaps because I wanted so desperately for things to be different for her than they were for me. For all of these reasons, Mary Kathryn brought me to the very center of my heart, where my greatest fears and deepest love mingled in a turbulent pool.

My husband, Keven, was a quiet source of strength and stability. He never wavered in doing what he thought was best for me. He investigated all the medical issues I faced, became an expert, it seemed, in melanoma, and learned all he could about the potential treatments. He brought me to my doctors and he always traveled with me to specialists who were out of town. And he did all of that while maintaining his law practice and serving as president of Rhode Island's 1986 Constitutional Convention.

Meanwhile, he constantly tried to find ways of deflating the tension we both felt with his humor. As we would get into the car to see yet another doctor, Keven would say, "Well, Marlene, we're off to consult with one of the three monkeys: 'see no evil, hear no evil, and speak no evil.' Which one is it going to be today?"

Despite the enormity of my problems, Keven was always upbeat about the likelihood that I would survive. At least he was with me. While we drove to the doctor or sat in some coffee shop waiting for my lab results, he would assure me that some medical therapy would turn up and save me. Little did I know that he had profound doubts about whether or not I would survive. He even confided to a couple of friends that he was afraid I wouldn't pull through. He didn't see anything in medicine that would help me, he told his confidants, and didn't know where we could turn for help. Yet with me, he remained positive, which was another sign of his strength and his commitment to do all he could to help me. No matter what we encountered, he insisted that we would find a way, that we would somehow make it through this terrible crisis. His unrelenting support gave me more hope. I trusted his judgment. If he believed, then part of me believed, as well. His hope made me feel less isolated, less alone. His belief that I would get better somehow meant that he and I—our marriage—would continue. I had no strength, but he was strong, maybe strong enough for both of us. We were comrades in arms, struggling against a common enemy. And in a very real sense, I counted on him to believe, because in my extremely weakened condition, he became my lifeline, my tether to this world. No doubt Keven sensed this, which placed an even greater burden on him.

His quiet, supportive manner was how he showed me his love. Keven and I were never very good at expressing our feelings. At one time in our marriage we sought the counseling of our local priest, who, after listening to us describe our relationship, said that we were the type of couple that functioned best when we were doing things together. We were better at talking about our shared responsibilities as parents and providers than we were about our emotions. Our longest conversations tended to be about our schedules, and which one of us could be with the children that night. Remarkably, neither of us thought about our feelings very much.

Even before I got cancer, both of us were suffering enormously from the demands of our lives and especially our careers. Neither of us had time for ourselves, much less each other. We gave ourselves to the children and to our work and neglected our own personal needs, and those of our relationship, almost entirely. As our priest had so astutely observed, we experienced closeness by *doing* things together, rather than simply by *being* together in any real sense. Now life had given us a terrible crisis, and there was much to do.

CHAPTER 3

From Within the Darkness, a Tiny Light

Dying is a lonely journey. It is a walk deeper and deeper into isolation until finally you are gone. After a while, you understand why you are alone and why people don't want to associate with you anymore. You are a walking reminder of everyone's greatest fear. Part of how we endure life is by shutting out thoughts of death. How many of us want to think about our tenuous hold on our most precious possession—our very life? I didn't blame people who dropped me from their social circle now. I understood completely.

Social encounters were burdensome for me, as well, because many encounters with old friends were awkward now. People acted strangely around me. Some avoided me entirely. They'd see me in the checkout line at the grocery store and pretend not to notice me. Or they'd see me coming down the street and then cross the street before we intersected. They didn't know what to say to me. Besides, how many times can you say, "I am sorry that you're ill" or "I hope you're feeling better." Some of my friends were overly sympathetic. They strained to say the right things, to offer some hope, even when it was obvious they didn't believe their hopeful words for an instant. How could they? Just to look at

me was painful for many people. Still, people felt they had to
say something, and all they could think to say were things
like: "You'll pull through, Marlene. We've got the best medical
system in the world. What do your doctors say?"

"Well, they're not very optimistic," I sometimes replied.

"You've got to be optimistic, Marlene. Optimism is good for
the immune system. I have read about people who survived
cancer just by being optimistic. . . ."

Our culture detests unhappy endings. Somehow, stories of
mothers leaving their children before they are grown seem
un-American. We are a people who want to believe that even
in the midst of darkness, there is light, happiness, and meaning. We are masters of the silver lining, of turning lemons into
lemonade. Our whole medical system is a monument to
keeping people alive, even when they are long past saving.
We deny death, even when it is obvious and inevitable, even
when it appears in those closest to us. But in some very personal and fundamental way, I interpreted the reaction of my
old friends as a rejection of me.

I understood their reaction, at least intellectually. This is
how we stay young and vibrant, but it's also how we stay
naive and superficial, how we lose our appreciation for life,
and how we overlook the small moments of intimacy between ourselves and those we love. I especially longed for
people to accept and embrace me *now*. Even though I had
Keven, I still needed people outside my family who could just
be with me without expecting me to participate in some false
hope, an illusion that they needed more than I. I yearned for
people who were strong enough to hold me, to hold death,
without blinking or turning away. By rejecting me, they were
demonstrating their fear, and I had too much fear already. I
suppose I was looking for a nurturing community, one that
accepted death, and in their acceptance would help me to die
peacefully.

And then this prayer was answered in the person of Evelyn
Rachko, a little Irish lady in her mid-fifties, short, stout, and

strong in both body and spirit. Evelyn was an emergency room nurse. She had seen it all. But even more, she radiated with maternal care.

Evelyn had six children; her youngest daughter was a friend of Mary Kathryn's. Her husband, tall and thin, worked for the city. Evelyn was strong, very much her own person, and very upbeat. She had accepted life, it seemed to me; she didn't feel the need to change people, or the way things were.

She had no trouble looking me in the eye and asking me what I needed: "Groceries? Fine. Make a list."; "Let me take the children for a walk. You rest. We'll be back in an hour."; "I'll drive you to your appointment with the doctor."; "How are you today? Are you feeling weak? Would you like some food?"; "I brought you some soup today. I made it last night and thought, 'Marlene might like some of this.' "

This is how she was: direct and to the point. She entered my house, sized up what needed doing, and then started doing it. Sometimes, all I needed was a little company, someone to talk to. Other times, I needed someone to help me with a specific chore or errand or simply to help me straighten the house. She did it.

She reminded me of someone from "the old country," if you know what I mean. In the life of a village, people are born, they develop, suffer crises, are restored, grow old, and eventually die. The people of the village witness the whole of life and, to varying degrees, somehow learn to accept it. Evelyn had that kind of spirit. She seemed to hold and accept the whole of life—and she still managed to smile a lot. She had treated people with gunshot and knife wounds, broken bones and broken hearts; she had seen a lot of death and a lot of miraculous recoveries. She didn't flinch when she looked at me.

Evelyn visited me several times a week and gave me whatever she had time to give. She didn't attempt to escape the details of my dying. On the contrary, she entered my world and attempted to serve me in any way she could. Evelyn was a practicing Catholic and as far as she was concerned, my fate was in God's hands. She knew perfectly well that I was dying. But she knew even more that I needed help, which meant that I needed her. God sends such people to us, I thought, to remind us that we are never truly alone.

Evelyn's presence was a singular gift, it seemed to me. I did not see her in any larger terms. But in fact, events were taking place without my knowledge—or participation—that would awaken me to the web of life in which we all live.

My brother Albert Marcello, who is an environmental and health engineer for the state of Rhode Island, was listening to a talk show on the radio one night in April 1986. The host of the show had on a guest who claimed to be a psychic. At one point the show's host invited listeners to call in with their questions for her guest. Albert is a very practical guy—you don't end up as an engineer without being eminently practical—but he was so impressed with the woman he decided to call in and ask her if he could help me.

"My sister is very depressed," he said to the woman. "Is there anything I can do for her?"

"Your sister is ill, isn't she?" the woman asked.

"Yes, she's very ill. She has cancer," Albert told her.

"She's given up all hope," the woman said. "But she shouldn't. Tell her about macrobiotics. Many people are benefiting from using that diet. I believe your sister can be helped if she adopts a macrobiotic diet."

Albert had never heard the word macrobiotic before. He quickly got a pencil and paper and wrote it down. The next day he went to a bookstore, bought a book about macrobiotics, and then came immediately to my house. When he rang the bell and entered my foyer, he was obviously excited to see me.

"I've got something for you that I think is important," he said. With that, he handed me a book entitled *The Cancer Prevention Diet* by Michio Kushi.

I looked at the cover, read the title, and said, "Albert, I'm way beyond cancer prevention. I'm into cancer treatment."

"No, no," he said. "This book can help you now. It's going to show you how to get well. Read it, please. It's all about the cause of cancer, even the cause of melanoma. It also shows how you can use food to recover."

"Food, Al? How is food going to help me overcome cancer?"

"Please, read the book. It will explain everything," he said.

I looked at Al. He had so much love and hope on his face.

"Okay," I said. "I'll read the book tonight." With that, I embraced him. "I love you. Thank you."

Welcome to Wonderland

It's rare, I believe, to receive a gift that makes absolutely no sense to you, but that was the case with the gift of macrobiotics that my brother had given to me. At first, this book, *The Cancer Prevention Diet*, seemed as illogical and arbitrary as cancer itself. The whole notion that health was in any way connected with our diets was new to me. What could food possibly have to do with cancer? I thought. But that was the foundation of the macrobiotic philosophy: Food either causes health or illness, depending on what you eat.

The macrobiotic thesis was that humans evolved on, and are dependent upon, a plant-based diet composed of whole grains, fresh vegetables, beans, sea vegetables, and a variety of fermented foods. Cancer, Kushi maintained, is the result of the modern diet, rich in fat, cholesterol, processed grains, artificial ingredients, and sugar—a diet, he said, humans were never designed to eat. With the exception of small amounts of fish, the macrobiotic diet was essentially a vegetarian regimen.

In addition to this strange dietary approach was the macrobiotic philosophy of yin and yang, a philosophy that I would later understand was of Chinese origin. According to this philosophy, all reality is composed of opposites. Time, space, physical dimensions, and movement were all based on opposites, such as day and night, male and female, high and low, left and right, near and far, hot and cold, up and down. Like the positive and negative poles of a magnet, opposites attract, intermingle, and create something new. That new thing was essentially a state of balance, brought about by the interaction of the opposites. The philosophy was not unfamiliar to me. I had encountered Hegel's dialectic in college and remembered very well the essential point that thesis and antithesis collide to create a new thing, the synthesis.

The Chinese maintained that yin and yang are essentially forces that can be understand as opposite spirals. Yin is a centrifugal force, radiating outward. It brings about such characteristics as expansion, coolness, and moisture. It is also associated with the moon, the feminine, nighttime, and passivity. Yang, the centripetal force that spirals inward, creates contraction, heat, and dryness. It is associated with the sun, masculinity, daytime, and activity.

Yin and yang are everywhere in life, this theory states, constantly attracting, intermingling, and creating something new. They are the basis for creation in the material world. While these two forces are present in everything, they can be manipulated most directly for our benefit through our food.

Some foods are yin in nature. These include beans, vegetables, fruit, processed foods, soft and sweet dairy products (including ice cream, yogurt, and milk), sugar, chemicals, alcohol, and—in the extreme—drugs. Others are yang in nature. Animal foods, such as fish, chicken, eggs, hard cheese, and red meat, are all increasingly yang. Salt is extremely yang. Whole grains are said to be balanced.

Each food, depending on its yin or yang nature, will have a specific influence on the body. Yin foods, in general, affect the upper part of the body, because they create a rising and expansive energy. Yang foods tend to affect the lower part of the body, primarily because they have a downward and contracting influence. When too much yin foods are eaten, they create problems above the diaphragm and on the skin. When too many yang foods are eaten, they tend to affect organs below the diaphragm, such as the intestinal tract, kidneys, and sex organs.

Melanoma, the book said, was a combination of extremes of yin and yang. The cancer itself, Kushi maintained, is a combination of both a skin disease—which is caused by yin foods, such as sugar, fruit, and chemicals—and a disorder of the muscles and bones, which are affected by extremes of yang foods, such as meat, eggs, poultry, and hard dairy products.

I wasn't sure of the significance of all of this. When I asked myself what my dietary imbalance might be, my love of sugar, especially fudge, came immediately to mind. I ate a piece of fudge almost every night before bed. On the other hand, the three meals I ate each day were made up primarily of animal foods. I didn't eat many vegetables and I wasn't a salad lover.

But was my diet any different from anyone else's? Not really, I thought. The diets of everyone I knew were made up of the same extremes as mine. And who's to say that such foods were extremes? These were ordinary foods: meat, chicken, eggs, dairy products, and fudge, for crying out loud!

Before I put the book down, I skimmed some of the other chapters. I was ready to dismiss the whole thing, when the title of one chapter caught my eye: "Medically Terminal or Macrobiotically Hopeful?" In it, Kushi listed the factors he believed hindered a person's ability to overcome cancer with macrobiotics. The first was lack of gratitude, especially for the food. Many people who adopt macrobiotics have no appreciation for the food, or the philosophy. They fully intend to go back to their old ways the minute they get well again. In other words, the cancer has not taught them anything, Kushi maintained. They have no better understanding of themselves, their relationship with God, or their relationship with nature as a result of their disease.

The second factor was an inaccurate dietary practice; in other words, they didn't know how to maintain the diet properly and therefore could not use the food effectively to overcome their illness. The third was lack of will; people simply give up their will to live. (I could relate to that one.) The fourth was lack of family support. Kushi wrote about people who came to him with cancer, hoping to use macrobiotics to get well. When he asked them where their wives or husbands were, they answered that their spouse did not want to be involved in any sort of dietary change, and would not help cook the food for them. That saddened me. I thought of how much Keven had helped me; I was sure he would change his diet, if that's what I wanted.

The fifth factor was loss of natural healing ability. When supported by the right conditions, the body heals itself, Kushi maintained. Unfortunately, excessive amounts of chemotherapy and other medical treatments can destroy the body's natural abilities to heal, Kushi argued, which makes recovery impossible.

Spiritual awareness, which Kushi defined as an unwillingness to blame others, fate, or some outside force for one's disease, was the next most important factor in recovery. People who get well, he said, see macrobiotics as one of many gifts from the universe, or God. They see it as an important step on their path to healing. They have a reverent approach, not only to the diet, but to all of life. They are grateful for their illness and for the changes it has brought into their lives. As they get well, they feel closer to the source of life.

This was the only chapter that made any sense to me, though I could not explain why it had the ring of truth. I put the book down. On the whole, macrobiotics had little or no appeal to me, except for this little chapter of Kushi's book. The words in that chapter lingered. On some level, they suggested a certain underlying spiritual approach to life and to healing, which stirred something in me.

The following day my brother Albert called to ask what my reaction was to *The Cancer Prevention Diet*.

"I don't know, Albert," I told him. "I don't really believe that diet can cure my cancer."

"But it may help, Marlene," Albert said. "I really think you should try it. What have you got to lose? Look, there's a person in Providence who runs some kind of macrobiotic teaching center. It's called the East West Center. Her name is Eileen Shea. Why don't you call her and ask for more information?"

Out of love for my brother, and because he had gone to the trouble of finding this woman, I acquiesced to his request.

On the phone Eileen Shea was friendly and supportive. She listened to my story and then encouraged me to see a macrobiotic counselor, who could give me specific recommendations on how to use the diet to get well.

"Do you know anyone who does that kind of thing?" I asked.

"Yes," she said. "I have just the person you should see— Marc Van Cauwenberg. Marc's a medical doctor and also a macrobiotic consultant. He's at the Kushi Institute in Boston." With that, she gave me the number of the Kushi Institute. Five minutes later, I had an appointment to see Dr. Van Cauwenberg.

I had taken the first step into Wonderland, I realized. I felt some trepidation and a little exhaustion at the mere thought of macrobiotics. God, it seemed so odd, so completely foreign. *Ugh.* Hadn't I been through enough already?

Al insisted on going with me to Boston to meet Dr. Van Cauwenberg. "I got you into this, Marlene, I might as well go all the way," he said. My appointment with Dr. Van Cauwenberg was scheduled for April 30, 1986, at 2 P.M. at the Kushi Institute in Brookline Village, a little hamlet of Boston. I was not feeling good at all on the day we went. I felt weak and detached from myself, as if I were only half present. Al recalls that I was in a daze, but I appeared slightly angry that he was putting me through all of this, too. I certainly thought that there was absolutely nothing of value to be found in macrobiotics, and, yes, the trip seemed like a waste of time.

The Kushi Institute, the leading educational center for macrobiotics, was housed in a building that once was an old factory mill. Like many such buildings throughout New England, this mill had been abandoned when the factory went out of business, and had since been refurbished. Made of old brown brick, the building stood three stories. A tiny, almost claustrophobic foyer served as an entrance to a narrow wooden stairwell that led to the Kushi Institute, on the third floor. My first impressions were not positive. Al and I trudged up the well-worn stairs, opened a thick metal door, and entered a hallway. We took several cautious steps, opened a door to our right, and entered a large room, a loft with polished wood floors and large factory-type windows against the far wall. A long table stood to one side of the room, behind which sat two women who welcomed people who had come to see Dr. Van Cauwenberg. There was a doorway that led into an inner office, where I presumed Dr. Van Cauwenberg would be found. I was asked to fill out some forms; when I finished, we were escorted to an inner office where the doctor sat behind a desk.

When we entered, he got up quickly and hurried over to greet Al and me. He was tall and thin, with brown hair and a little brown mustache. His face was impressive for its sharp, intelligent features. His movements were quick and as he greeted us, he bowed his head and smiled gleefully, as if he had just heard a humorous joke. "Please," he said, as he pointed to two chairs that sat opposite his desk. As we took our seats, a young woman entered the cubicle and sat down, as well, with some forms in her hands. "She will take notes and give them to you when you leave," Dr. Van Cauwenberg said.

I explained my condition. After I had said as much as my strength allowed, I sat back in my chair, exhausted. The effort drained me of all my reserves and now I didn't have the strength to hold up any pretenses of civility. As far as I was concerned, this trip and the effort I just expended in explaining my condition had already been something of a rip-off. I did nothing to hide my negativity and my suspicion of macrobiotics and Dr. Van Cauwenberg.

Dr. Van Cauwenberg looked at me and said, "You're very sick."

A sharp, impolite retort jumped into my mouth, but I stifled it before I uttered the words. Instead, I sat there and looked at him as if he were a foolish child.

He then got up and gave me an examination unlike any I had had to that point. He looked into my eyes, asking me to look left, right, up, and down. He examined my face very carefully, and then my arms, especially the insides of my forearms. He then asked me to remove my shoes and, when I did, turned his attention to my feet.

"You must be very strict on the diet if you are to recover," he said.

With that, he outlined the kind of macrobiotic diet I was to eat.

"You must not have any raw foods," he began. "None. Okay? Every food I recommend must be cooked. Grains can be pressure-cooked or boiled; beans can be boiled, or sometimes pressure-cooked with a grain. Vegetables can be boiled or steamed."

As he spoke, I finally realized that he had an accent. Because I was educated in France and familiar with many European accents, I recognized it as either Dutch or Flemish. I later learned he was Belgian and his accent indeed was Flemish.

"You must avoid extremes," he said. There was that word again, I thought.

"No red meat," Dr. Van Cauwenberg was saying. "No

chicken, eggs, or dairy foods, and no sugar, no white flour products, no synthetic chemicals or food additives.

"All your food must be fresh and you should cook it every day if you can. Leftover foods, especially dry foods, have no vitality left," he said. Somehow, I understood that, even though, at the time, I could not articulate why. It made sense to me that dried-out foods had no vitality, or life, in them.

"Brown rice. It should be soft and moist. Have soft grains, such as rice, whole oats, barley, millet. Season with a little miso, or *gomashio,* chopped scallions, or other condiments.

"For breakfast, have soft grains. A little *amasake* is okay if used sparingly."

As he spoke, the young woman dutifully took down everything he said. Good, I thought, because I have no idea what many of these foods were; nor could I remember their names.

"Every day at breakfast have miso soup and seaweed together in the same bowl." He chuckled, I presumed, at the lengths he was going to instruct me. He was not at all condescending, however.

I cannot say that I was so polite. "How do you expect me to eat seaweed?" I asked. "Why do I have to eat all of these strange foods?"

"The diet you have followed is responsible for giving you cancer," Dr. Van Cauwenberg said. "If you continue to eat that way, you soon will be dead."

"I don't get it," I retorted. "What's wrong with my diet?"

"You eat too much sugar, especially chocolate, and too much red meat, eggs, and dairy foods," he said. I was momentarily stunned.

"How do you know I eat too much chocolate?" I inquired.

"I can see it on your face," he said. "All this darkness on your cheeks, especially these patches of brown"—he pointed to the area around my mouth, under my eyes, and cheeks—"that's sugar coming out, and your face tells me that you especially like chocolate."

"Why can't I just give up chocolate and eat more vegetables?" I said.

"Because your diet is imbalanced. That's what we are doing with the diet I have given you: restoring balance to your body so that you can heal yourself. Also, your current diet is loaded with poisons that are killing you," Dr. Van Cauwenberg said. "Have you ever eaten a whole grain, such as a bowl of brown rice or some barley, in your entire life?"

"No, I was raised on steak and tomato sauce. It was good enough for my parents and their parents; why shouldn't it be good enough for me!"

"Look at the results of your diet and lifestyle," he said. "It has led to cancer. That's why you have to change." Dr. Van Cauwenberg said this with great equanimity, even with a little smile on his lips.

I went on questioning him in an aggressive manner. It was as if I was trying to find some hole in the system so that I could reveal it as a fraud. Finally I looked over at Al, who was clearly upset.

"Marlene, listen to Dr. Van Cauwenberg," he said, and with that, he got up from his chair and left the room. I didn't know where he was going. Only later did he tell me that he left the room because I had become intolerably rude to a person who was trying to help me.

Once outside the office, Al stood and prayed to my father. "Dad, I know you're up there. Will you come down here and shake up your daughter because she's not listening." Suddenly the sun came out and it bathed the entire office area. Al was stunned. At that point he came back into the room.

Marc was still instructing me on how to eat. "Eat scallions and onions in the morning, as well," Marc was saying. "*Mochi* helps to provide strength and more endurance. It will give you energy. Have that for breakfast, two times a week.

"You can have one piece of sourdough bread per day, but it

must be steamed first. Use it plain or in soup. Avoid all oily butter from nuts. No fruit spreads, no soy margarine. All out! Avoid raisins, fruit. No deep frying of any foods. Use very little oil for sauté.

"Eat steamed greens at breakfast. Avoid barley malt and rice syrup, at least for the moment.

"For lunch and dinner, not so watery cooking as for breakfast. Use lighter grain for lunch, especially millet, corn, noodles. Eat *udon* noodles. Make your noodles with vegetables sometimes, like vegetable noodle soup.

"Try to make a fresh lunch every day, but sometimes you can reheat leftovers.

"Avoid tomatoes, eggplant, lettuce, potato, zucchini, spinach, and red beets. Avoid also alcohol and beer.

"You may have soup two times a day, if you like. Eat beans—*azuki,* chickpeas, lentils, black beans. Tofu is okay. Tempeh, not so much at the moment. Maybe once every two weeks.

"Sea vegetables. Eat *wakame* in soup and *kombu* in beans. That's enough for now. Leafy greens and a variety of vegetables." He then listed many vegetables, including collard greens, kale, mustard greens, broccoli, cabbage, squash, carrots, rutabaga, turnips, and daikon radish.

"*Seitan.*" He must have seen the utterly baffled look on my face, because for the first time he actually defined one of the many foreign foods he had mentioned. "That's wheat gluten. Cook *seitan* with vegetables or by itself. You can fry in a little oil.

"Avoid seafood or shellfish for the moment. As for your liquid, you can have water and *bancha* tea, a little *yannoh,* or grain coffee, and *Mu* tea #9 or #16.

"Avoid snacks between meals, but if you desire, eat a little rice cakes with bean spread, such as chickpea spread, or lentil spread.

"Rice bread or corn bread is okay, as long as it is prepared without chemicals, dairy foods, or eggs. All pasta is okay as long as it is made from whole grains. Buckwheat noodles, called *soba,* are okay, too.

"Use *gomashio* as a condiment. *Gomashio* is sesame seeds and a small amount of sea salt. Warm up sauerkraut and use with bread and other grains. You must chew all your food thoroughly. Get some exercise every day. Just walking is okay. Don't exert yourself too much."

He then sat back in his chair and looked at me, as if sizing me up. He said nothing for a time. "You can get all of these foods at Erewhon, right up the street from here," he said, mentioning a nearby natural foods store in Brookline Village. "You can buy cookbooks right here. You should also get cooking lessons. Do you have any questions?"

I was so overwhelmed and dumbfounded I could not think of anything to ask him. Where do I begin, I thought. Nothing about this food or way of life is familiar or makes any sense to me. My mind was a blank.

"Do you think this can help Marlene? Can she recover?" Al asked.

"Yes, if she does it properly and to the letter. She must be absolutely strict." He looked at me and said, "After a while, when you get your health back, you can widen your diet, but not before you show real progress."

Dr. Van Cauwenberg got up from his chair and walked over to me and shook my hand. He then shook Al's hand and gave both of us a very happy, warm smile. None of my rude behavior had affected him in the slightest. He was as happy at the end of our meeting as he was when we walked in.

With that, the session was over. We had been there about an hour, and when we left, our heads were spinning. As we drove back to Providence, I wrestled within myself over what to do. "The whole thing is crazy, Al," I said more than once. "I think they've all gone nuts over there."

"I don't know, Marlene," Al said. "Maybe they're right about some things."

We drove for a long time in silence. When we got home, I

went into the kitchen, sat down at my table, and rested. Then
I got up and looked at my cupboards: Canned soups, boxed
meals, cereals, and bags of sugar stared back at me, all of
them packaged in garish colors. I opened the refrigerator:
cartons of milk and eggs, sticks of butter, wedges of cheese,
steaks, bacon, chicken, cakes, and whole armies of processed
foods. In the freezer: ice cream and meat.

Nothing looked the same to me now. For some reason
these foods looked unhealthy to me, and the following day
my meals tasted unhealthy. I didn't know what to do. *The
Cancer Prevention Diet* and my meeting with Dr. Marc Van
Cauwenberg had thrown me into conflict.

I couldn't believe that the macrobiotic food could really
help me, but I admitted to myself that something was pulling
me in that direction. Could this food really help me? I wondered.

The Crossing

Two days after I had seen Marc Van Cauwenberg, my
brother Al dropped over to our house unexpectedly. He was
carrying a big bag of groceries. He held the bag with such
pride that you might have thought he was carrying a new
baby.

"I bought you some things," Al announced, almost gleefully. Inside the bag was an assortment of vegetables and
grains. I immediately made out bunches of leafy greens and
carrots. There was also a bag containing brown rice and another containing seaweed.

"Why did you do that?" I asked.

"Well, I thought you needed some help getting started," he
said, clearly happy with himself. What was that expression
on his face? Why did he seem to be taking such pleasure in
my new diet? The answer was obvious: He was proud that he
had introduced me to this new way of life. What was clear, as

well, was that he absolutely believed in the power of this food to help me overcome cancer. Any skepticism he might have had was gone after meeting Dr. Van Cauwenberg. As he stood there, helpful and proud, I could not help but feel my heart swell.

"Thank you," I said, with a laugh. "You're so sweet. But I don't even know what to do with these foods. I'm not even sure I'm going to do it, Al."

"Marlene, I think you should do it. I really do."

"It's all so foreign, Al. I don't know if I can do it."

"Call the woman at the macrobiotic center in town," Al said. He was referring to Eileen Shea. "She'll help you. She gives cooking classes. She'll teach you how to prepare all this stuff."

"I'll think about it," I said.

"Promise me you'll think very hard about adopting the macrobiotic diet," Al said.

"I promise I'll think about it," I said.

After Al left, I opened my cupboards and refrigerator and looked at my foods again. In an instant I had decided. I went outside and brought my garbage can into the kitchen and started throwing out everything in my cupboards and everything in the refrigerator.

I made such a racket that Keven came running into the kitchen and looked at me aghast.

"I'm going to do it," I said.

CHAPTER 4

Entering the World of Macrobiotics

I stood in the middle of my kitchen and wondered, What have I done? Somehow, it felt as if my old life had been packed up and thrown into the garbage, as well. My cupboards and refrigerator were bare, and I felt it in my soul. I cleaned the kitchen, as much as my strength would allow. I always felt an underlying weakness and I tired quickly. Yet, I felt vaguely exhilarated, too. I was starting a new life. How long it lasted would depend on whether or not the macrobiotic diet could help me overcome cancer or, short of that, slow the progress of my disease. But embracing macrobiotics—which meant accepting the philosophy and preparing and eating the food—would not be easy. Just thinking about going out and buying the foods Marc Van Cauwenberg had recommended was daunting. Suddenly I felt deeply tired. I slumped into a chair. What had I got myself into?

And then it hit me: What have I got my family into? I realized that I had thrown out the foods *they* were used to eating, as well. I looked at my cupboards again and wondered if there was enough food for their dinner that night. No. I better go out and buy food, and it might as well be macrobiotic foods.

I telephoned Eileen Shea and told her about my meeting with Dr. Van Cauwenberg. She suggested that I bring the list of foods to the center so that we could go over them together. That afternoon I went to the East West Center at DePasquale Square in Providence and talked to Eileen.

The center was located in an old storefront in the Italian section of Providence. The main room was small—perhaps twenty-five feet square—with a little kitchen in the back. There was a large rectangular opening in the wall—a kind of open window—that provided a waist-high countertop and allowed people to look into the kitchen, perfect for the cooking classes that Eileen said she gave here. The linoleum floors were well-worn. About ten or twelve small tables for four were arranged throughout the room. Tall, standing plants had been placed in the corners of the room, and a few more plants hung in the windows. Curtains framed the sides of the windows, allowing the sun to come pouring into the room. A strong aroma of food hung in the air. The smell was foreign to me, but not at all unpleasant. I could not get over how cozy and homey the place was. The small size made it intimate, and the smells and plants gave it life. This was an old storefront that obviously had been transformed with care.

Eileen was clearly in her element, moving about the room with an unconscious familiarity that one associates with being at home. She was about five feet six inches, strong-boned and attractive, with high cheekbones, brown eyes and brown hair. She was married and had four children, I would later learn. She was relaxed, open, and patient. She gave you the feeling that when she sat down and looked at you, she had really landed and was fully present. There was nothing distracting her from giving you all of her attention. And yet she was also light and very humble. She smiled and laughed easily. Her personality seemed to reach out from her and embrace you. As I would later learn, she took everyone who entered this place under her wing, showering them with support and love. Clearly, the East West Center of Providence was her mission.

We went over Marc Van Cauwenberg's directions together, point by point. What an assortment of strange substances they were to me! She explained the importance of each of the foods he had recommended, starting with the whole grains, including brown rice, millet, oats, barley, corn, wheat, and buckwheat. Whole grains were important, she said, because they were loaded with complex carbohydrates, which would give me energy. They contained lots of important vitamins and minerals to strengthen my body's healing mechanisms. Grains also are rich sources of fiber, which help digestion and the elimination of toxins. Grains were the foods closest to being balanced between yin and yang, Eileen said. She explained a little about yin and yang, but the words and the concepts still baffled me. I wasn't ready to embrace them. She then turned to miso, a fermented soybean paste that is used to make soups and sauces. Miso aids digestion, Eileen said. It restores friendly bacteria in the intestinal tract and strengthens the blood and immune function. Tamari and shoyu, also made from fermented soybeans, were liquid sauces, like soy sauce, only of far superior quality, containing no chemicals or artificial ingredients. Like miso, they restored healthy bacteria and supported digestion. They also alkalized the intestines and blood, which Eileen said was important to supporting the body's healing forces. Then there was daikon radish, a long white radish not unlike a carrot, which, Eileen said, would break up tumors and fat deposits and strengthen my kidneys. We then discussed the seaweeds, dulse, *arame, hijiki, kombu,* and *wakame.* Seaweed, she said, was among the richest sources of minerals and vitamins in the food supply. *Hijiki* contains 1,500 milligrams of calcium in a single cup.

"You're going to need cooking classes and help preparing the food, Marlene," she said. "At first, there's some adjustment to the flavors because they're so different from what you're used to eating. Believe it or not, you're going to actually prefer eating macrobiotic food before too long." That seemed impossible!

As we neared the end of our discussion, Eileen asked me an odd question, "Do you have a gas stove?"

"No, I have an electric stove," I answered. "Why do you ask?"

"Marlene, if you want to live, you'll get a gas stove," she said. Her words fairly shocked me. She then explained that macrobiotic healing was based on the idea that food is energy and that energy is the basis for life. Every living thing possesses its own energetic qualities, but so, too, do most inanimate objects. When a person says that they sense a person's personality or character, they are actually sensing his or her energetic nature, or the nature of the person's energy that lives inside of them. Is the energy balanced, peaceful, and open, or is it aggressive, closed, or even violent? All of us sense these and many other characteristics in others, as well as in situations. A characteristic energy—what you might call the essence or nature of a certain thing—is contained within every living thing, every object, and every situation. Fire has a powerful, healing energy that is conveyed to food when fire is used in cooking. We consume that energy when we eat food that has been prepared over a flame. On the other hand, electricity conveys a weak, chaotic energy that is transferred into the food and then into our cells. That disorderly energy from electricity slows the healing process and may even prevent it.

Besides, she said with a smile, the food tastes better when you cook it on a gas range.

I didn't know where to begin to debate what seemed to me to be another irrational tenet of macrobiotics. I was too weak to argue anyway. I took a deep breath and said that I would look into getting a gas stove.

On my way home from Eileen, I stopped off at a little natural foods store in Providence, called Golden Sheaf, and bought the macrobiotic staples that Marc and Eileen had recommended. I also bought two new macrobiotic books—a cookbook by Aveline Kushi, entitled *The Complete Guide to Macrobiotic Cooking,* and *The Book of Macrobiotics,* by Michio Kushi. I then went home and called up a local appliance store and ordered a gas stove. Looking back, I realize now that I was doing more than just accommodating Eileen Shea. I was throwing my faith entirely into this new way of life.

I was struck by how different the world of macrobiotics was from my old life of business, finance, and stress. Even though I was on a leave of absence from my job, I still called in almost every day to check with my assistant, Jeannine, on how business was going and to discuss any latest issue that had arisen. Jeannine was smart and bubbly. She knew how grave my situation was and constantly reassured me that all was well and that I needn't worry about anything.

"When you get back, Marlene, you'll see that nothing has changed," she assured me. "It's the same rat race. Just the names and faces have been changed to protect the guilty—there are no innocents around here, you know that." Jeannine always had a way of reassuring me that I still had a place at my job.

"Thanks, Jeannine. But you take care of yourself," I said. "Get away from that place whenever you can. I'm seeing more and more how my lifestyle really contributed to my getting sick."

"Yeah, I hear you, Marlene," Jeannine said. "Thanks. But you take care now and don't worry about this crazy place."

Already, macrobiotics was changing how I saw my old life. The philosophy of macrobiotics contrasted so starkly with the values that supported my old lifestyle that I couldn't help but have a new perspective on my old way of living.

A Disastrous Beginning

After a nap I awoke feeling a bit stronger and eager to start eating a macrobiotic meal. I went into the kitchen, emptied the bags of groceries on my table, and began to fill my cupboards. I still didn't know how to prepare most of the foods I had purchased, but I had been cooking for more than twenty years. What could be so difficult?

That night I prepared my first macrobiotic meal. I wanted to keep it simple, so I boiled brown rice, chopped and steamed kale and carrots, and also boiled a couple of cups of *hijiki* seaweed. My kitchen was filled with an odd smell, which did nothing for my appetite. When Keven came home that night, he walked into the kitchen and asked, "What is that smell?"

"That's dinner, Keven," I said, smiling. "I'm making our first macrobiotic meal."

"Are you supposed to eat it or paint the driveway with it?" Keven asked.

"We'll see," I said, with a little laugh.

Keven chuckled, as well, and left the room. There was always Chinese take-out, in case the meal failed, I thought.

The kids helped me set the table and we all sat down to our macrobiotic meal. It was a disaster. The rice and vegetables were bland and virtually tasteless. "Can't we put some butter or something on this food, Mom? Maybe it needs some soy sauce?" Christopher asked. The other children moaned. "Mom!?" Nothing could have prepared us for the seaweed, however. "*Oooooo!*" everyone moaned. "It's terrible! I'm not eating that stuff."

They were right. It was wretched. It had to be the worst-tasting substance I had ever put in my mouth. I wouldn't even paint my driveway with it. Pretty soon the children were all asking that we go out to dinner or get some food delivered. Eventually Keven agreed to take them to McDonald's.

"Do you want to go, Marlene?" Keven asked. "We can start the diet another day."

"No, thanks," I said. "Maybe the food tastes bad because I don't know how to cook it yet. Eileen said it would eventually taste good."

"Well, maybe she's right," he said, trying to sound hopeful. With that, he joined the children who were urging him to hurry up. "We're starved," they were saying. "Let's go, Dad."

I sat at the table, alone. How could I eat this every day? My heart sank. If this was my path to health, could I walk it? I ate some more rice and vegetables, threw out the seaweed, and cleaned the dishes. I just don't know how to prepare the food yet, I told myself. Eileen did not strike me as the kind of person who would lie about the food tasting good eventually.

Tired and depressed, I went into the living room, put my feet up, and started to read Aveline Kushi's cookbook. Aveline is the wife of author Michio Kushi. I perused some recipes, but everything sounded so foreign that I couldn't tell whether the food would be good or not. I then turned to the book's introduction, which gave a short presentation on the macrobiotic food and the philosophy. Every time I confronted macrobiotics, it seemed to shock me in some way: the ideas, the food, the way of life. Was this madness, or had I really stumbled upon something worth doing?

Of course, the idea that was most incredible to me was that the macrobiotic diet and lifestyle could cure my cancer. It was the macrobiotic contention that the food we eat each day creates our blood and determines the body's capacity to resist and overcome disease. Food provides the nutrients the body needs to restore its own self-healing powers. Given the right conditions—namely, a balanced diet and lifestyle—the body itself can restore health. That was the essence of the philosophy, insofar as I could make out, but from there it seemed to spiral into every aspect of life.

The whole notion of balance was unlike anything I was accustomed to. Contrary to how the U.S. Department of

Agriculture defined balance—the food pyramid with its daily portions of red meat, dairy food, grains, and vegetables—the macrobiotic philosophy understood balance as the harmony between two cosmic forces, yin and yang. The food we eat was the primary tool for creating this balance, which itself was the basis for health or illness. Excessive consumption of either yin foods or yang foods resulted in imbalance and illness. For example, too many yin foods and substances, such as refined-flour products, artificial ingredients, sugar, alcohol, and drugs, drained the nervous system of minerals and caused scattered thinking and erratic behavior. People who consumed such products became forgetful, unable to concentrate, in a word, "spacey." Eventually they became weak and ill. Yin diseases often manifested in the upper part of the body, above the diaphragm, and on the skin. Bronchitis, sinus trouble, stroke, and brain tumors, for example, all resulted, at least in part, from the overconsumption of yin foods. Excess yang foods, such as red meat, chicken, fish, and salt, caused people to become too narrowly focused, overly ambitious, aggressive, and tense. They sought to control life too much. In the extreme, many could become selfish, stubborn, and greedy. They often got heart disease, lung cancer, and illnesses affecting organs and tissues below the diaphragm, such as digestive or reproductive disorders. It was clear that both extremes led to disaster.

A diet balanced in yin and yang was made up of whole grains, fresh vegetables, beans, fruit, and fish. This, the macrobiotic philosophy maintained, gave rise to strong, mineral-rich blood that was resistant to illness. It created a balanced view of life, as well. People who ate such a diet tended to be more emotionally secure and open. They enjoyed mental clarity, abundant energy, and good health.

As implausible as these ideas seemed to my rational mind, I nonetheless held on to them for dear life. It wasn't easy. Everything about the macrobiotic philosophy and way of life seemed strange and irrational to me at first. I looked again at some of the recipes. They didn't sound so bad, I told myself. Maybe Eileen is right. I just need time to get used to the food and to learn how to prepare it. I needed cooking classes, as Eileen had said. But I doubted my ability to turn these foods into delicious meals. I needed help. And then it struck me: I should hire a cook who is familiar with these foods. There must be lots of people in the Providence area who know something about this type of cooking.

The next day I put an ad in the *Providence Journal*: "Wanted: cook to help Mother prepare Oriental-style foods at my home." I included my telephone number in the ad and prayed that the right person would come along.

That week, I continued to struggle with the macrobiotic foods while my husband and children ate out most nights. My meals consisted of boiled brown rice, some steamed leafy greens, and boiled carrots. That was the extent of the cooking I could do. I did not dare attempt the seaweed again. Nor did I feel sufficiently confident to use the pressure cooker to prepare brown rice. Boiling my food made it very bland. My meals were essentially tasteless, as far as I was concerned. I couldn't eat this way for very long, I realized, but for now I would have to persevere.

My children reacted to my nightly dinners with a mixture of pity and confusion. "Why are you eating this way, Mom?" Mary Kathryn asked me.

"Because I believe it will make me feel better," I told her.

"It didn't make me feel better when I ate that food," she answered.

"I know, honey, but maybe Mommy doesn't know how to cook this food very well yet. It's new and different to me. I have to learn how to make it so that it's really delicious. Maybe then even you and your brothers will like it, too."

"Okay, but can we go out for dinner again tonight?"

I couldn't help laughing. "Yes," I said. "Your dad will take you out."

A Community Gathering

On Friday night of that week, Keven and I went to the East West Center to eat dinner and meet some of the people who were part of the macrobiotic community, which numbered a couple of hundred people in the Greater Providence area. Once a month one of the macrobiotic teachers from Boston would come to the center to lecture. When that happened, anywhere from twenty-five to forty people would show up.

The macrobiotic community of Providence was made up of a wide diversity of people, and equally wide assortment of ages. Though there were a few young singles and married couples, some with children, the majority were middle aged and older, most of them professionals.

Much to my surprise, Eileen had a twin sister, Elaine, who also worked at the center. Together they prepared and served the meals at the center. They also did some cooking classes together, though I was informed that Eileen did most of the teaching.

Keven and I took seats at one of the tables and pretty soon were joined by a man whose name was Tom Marron. Inevitably we started talking about how we came to macrobiotics, and Tom volunteered that he was using macrobiotics to overcome his cancer. He had malignant melanoma, Clark's Level III, which had spread to his lymph nodes. I was in shock. "That's what I am suffering from," I said. "How are you doing?"

At that point, Tom told Keven and me his remarkable story. Tom, a professional recruiter, was diagnosed with malignant melanoma three years earlier at the age of thirty-seven. A one-inch incision removed the cancerous mole on his upper left arm. Five months later, doctors removed a large cancerous tumor and a string of lymph nodes from Tom's armpit. The tumor, which had been growing steadily, was cancerous. There were numerous other growths throughout his body, as well. At this point doctors recommended radiation and chemotherapy, though they admitted to Tom that there was no cure for malignant melanoma and that they could not hold out much hope for his survival.

Tom decided not to undergo any further treatment, but instead adopted macrobiotics after reading a book entitled *Recalled By Life*. The book detailed Dr. Anthony Sattilaro's use of the macrobiotic diet to overcome prostate cancer, which had spread throughout his body. Dr. Sattilaro was president of Methodist Hospital in Philadelphia when he became sick. His story, which was also reported in *The Saturday Evening Post* and *Life* magazines, became a bestseller.

Shortly after adopting macrobiotics, Tom began to change his life radically. Everything in his life, it seemed, was wrong at this point. His job, which required long hours of commuting and offered only a straight commission on his work, was a constant source of stress. His marriage had been bad for many years. And his lifestyle was, in many ways, ruining his health. The first thing he did upon starting macrobiotics was quit his job. He supported himself with the money he had saved and began studying the macrobiotic philosophy and diet in Boston. He read numerous other books on health, including Norman Cousins's book *Anatomy of an Illness*, and Norman Vincent Peale's *The Power of Positive Thinking*. He used visualization techniques to improve his attitudes toward life and began to pray faithfully each day. He exercised daily. All of these practices transformed his life, but there was still a major issue lingering, which he had to resolve. At the center of his problems, Tom realized, was a marriage that just wasn't working. Eventually he and his wife decided to separate, and Tom took a room at Eileen Shea's house. Eileen cooked for him and gave him cooking lessons. At that point Tom's health started to make a rapid recovery.

One year later, doctors performed an array of tests—including a complete physical examination, blood tests, and X rays—and could find no sign of cancer anywhere in his body. But even before doctors confirmed that he was better, Tom knew deep inside that he had overcome his disease. (At the time of this writing, in the summer of 1999, Tom Marron remains in good health and cancer-free.)

"Macrobiotics was my foundation," Tom told Keven and me that night. "It was absolutely essential to my recovery. But I used a lot of other approaches to help myself, too," he said. "I kept looking for the answers, and new doors kept opening up for me. I had to transform my entire life in order to get well."

Tom's story was like a life preserver that had been thrown to me from a passing ship. I was lost in the water, with little hope that I had any chance of survival, when suddenly, as if from out of nowhere, he arrived at my table and gave me hope. I could have hugged him right there, even though I didn't know him. It could be done, he was saying. Here was living proof. I had to know more.

"But, Tom, didn't you find that this macrobiotic way of life is a bit, well, strange," I said, trying not to sound disrespectful. "At times I don't know what to believe."

"Oh, definitely, Marlene," Tom said. "Actually, I had read *Recalled By Life* about eight months before I was diagnosed with cancer. When I first read that book, the whole thing sounded bizarre to me. Nothing made sense. But after I was diagnosed in May of 1983, I read the book again and this time the whole thing made sense to me. I couldn't put that book down. A lot of it has to do with what you are ready for, what you're ready to understand and embrace.

"When I first started macrobiotics, I started to lose weight, which made everyone around me think that the diet was making the cancer worse. But then I went to Boston and started studying with the teachers up there and they told me that losing weight at the beginning of the diet wasn't bad, that I would be eliminating a lot of poisons and waste products from my body and that I would lose some weight in the process.

"By the time I moved into Eileen Shea's house, I was yellow and had lumps and bumps all over my body," Tom continued. "I was in terrible shape. But after two weeks of eating her food and being out of my house and away from my marriage, I was fifty percent better. All the lumps in my body were reduced by half. I knew then that I had found the right path. But you have to keep going, keep transforming aspects of your life that are the source of your imbalances and disease.

"In November 1984 doctors at Dana Farber Cancer Institute in Boston told me that I was well, that there was no sign of cancer in my body. They called it a miracle. They didn't know what to make of me."

Tom's words resonated deep inside me. I knew now that it was possible. I also knew that there was a long road ahead, and a lot for me to do.

With that, the meal was served. Silverware was available in a tray near the kitchen, but to my amazement, most people took chopsticks instead of forks, spoons, and knives. Keven and I were not ready for chopsticks.

The first thing that impressed me about Eileen's meal was the rich color. The food looked vibrant and very much alive. The leafy greens—I recognized the collards—and the carrots were bright green and orange. A white sauce—made from tofu, with flecks of scallion—covered some of the greens and carrots. The rice, which Tom said had been pressure-cooked, was the color of bamboo. A small mound of black turtle beans sat next to a lump of *arame* seaweed, which was black satin with brown highlights. A few yellow pickles—slices of pickled daikon radish—were arrayed next to the rice. Served with the meal was a bowl of miso soup, which was light brown. Swimming in the soup were small sheafs of *wakame* seaweed and a few pieces of sliced scallions.

I suddenly realized that the vegetables I had prepared at home clearly had been overcooked. But that had always been the case, no matter where I ate them, or who prepared them. Vegetables were an afterthought in my life. No one I knew had ever taken them seriously, or actually thought of them as an important part of the meal, much less a medicinal part of the meal.

I tried the soup, which—to my surprise—was not at all bad. It was salty-flavored, even briny, thanks to the seaweed, but pleasant. It was warming and seemed to strengthen me a bit. Contrary to my own meal, I did not find the seaweed in the soup at all repulsive, perhaps because the flavor of the soup masked any distinct taste of the seaweed. Next I tried the rice. Pressure-cooked rice, I quickly discovered, was so different from boiled rice, which is so watery and bland. Eileen had prepared the rice to perfection, it seemed to me. Each piece had its own integrity, yet it was soft and rich. The rice had a nutty flavor, which when chewed extensively—I had taken Mark Van Cauwenberg's advice to heart—yielded a sweet flavor that was delicious. The greens and carrots were pulpy and mild-tasting, but the sauce enhanced them considerably.

Finally, I tried the *arame* seaweed. I put a little in my mouth and immediately my palate said, "No. Ugh." It was altogether too foreign, too slimy, and repugnant. I swallowed quickly and went for the beans, which were rich, soft, and luscious. They overwhelmed the flavor of the seaweed.

Except for the seaweed, which would take some getting used to, the meal was far more delicious than I ever expected. I looked over at Keven and could tell that he, too, was enjoying the meal. In some odd and unexpected way I felt my life supported. I almost wanted to cry. I could do this, I said to myself. I could eat this way. Such gratitude as I had not felt in a long time welled up inside me.

CHAPTER 5

Learning the Power of the Food

I had been in counseling off and on since 1983. In the spring of 1986 I resumed the counseling with my counselor, Will Parnum. I needed professional help to cope with my fear of death and the pain of leaving my children. Once a week I entered his office and felt safe to unburden myself of all my fears, of how every cramp or twinge of pain brought a sudden heightened awareness of my disease. No physical discomfort or pain was innocent. There was no such thing as indigestion, or a benign muscle ache. Every form of discomfort, I was convinced, arose from the movement of the cancer inside me. Every pain awakened me to its presence and its exact location in my body. It was as if I had an evil life-form living inside of me, consuming and destroying me. I wanted to be ignorant of its presence; I wanted to forget it was ever there.

Now and then, for a few minutes or an hour, I did manage to forget. During these respites, my life almost felt normal. I didn't think of death at all. Instead, I was taken up by the need to pick up the kids at a certain hour, or by the fact that I had to run to the grocery store.

The instant I became conscious of myself, I would awaken

to the shadow that oppressed me. At that moment, I would suddenly realize that I had just spent the last few minutes free from fear, that for a short while I had been distracted by the salutary little details of life. Thank God for those little details, those precious little distractions that gave me back my life, I sometimes thought. But my awareness would inevitably return, and with it the fear of death.

I came to Will Parnum to talk about all of the many fears I faced during the week. Not surprisingly, that fear led to deeper issues about my work, my relationship with Keven and, most of all, with myself.

On the Monday morning, following the Friday night macrobiotic dinner, all three of these conflicts emerged in Parnum's office. Will had asked me a seemingly simple question: "How do you react when your work becomes demanding, or you experience conflict in your marriage?" The first answer that came to mind was, simply, "I get tense."

"Where do you experience that tension?" Will asked.

"Everywhere," I said.

"By everywhere, do you mean throughout your body?"

"Yes, but especially in my stomach area and shoulders," I said.

"Why don't you point to the place in your stomach where you feel that tension," Will asked.

I pointed to the area just below my solar plexus.

"Isn't that where your cancer was found?" Will said.

"Yes," I said. "It's where I had the operation, too, to remove part of my small intestine."

"Do you feel there's any connection," he asked.

"I don't know, but I am feeling that there must be," I said.

"When you bring your awareness to that place where you had the operation, what associations come up for you?"

I paused for a few moments while I attempted to feel the place where Will had directed my consciousness. "I feel wounded there, like I'm hurt," I said.

Will was silent now. He was waiting. I concentrated some more, and suddenly I couldn't hold back the tears. I began sobbing and shaking.

"What are you feeling?" Will asked.

Through my tears, I blurted out, "I feel my whole body crying. My whole body is like a little child, crying and calling out for attention, for love."

"Have you neglected your body?" Will asked.

I reached for the tissue box, which sat on an end table near my chair, and wiped the tears from my eyes and face. "Yes," I said. "I think I've neglected my body for a very long time."

"Why have you done that?" Will asked.

"I've always had a lot of guilt about my body," I said. "I guess I associate bodily pleasures with some kind of sin or something. I was only nine-and-a-half when I got my period and right away older women began telling me that I must stay away from boys from now on. I felt marked from that moment on, as if I had done something bad, or there was something bad about me. To this day I feel an inner conflict about my bodily functions and needs."

"Maybe you're having trouble with intimacy—intimacy with yourself, intimacy with your wounded body, and with others," Will suggested. "I think it's time to really start to care for yourself, especially your body, wouldn't you say? I mean, it seems as if you have rejected your body in a way."

"Yea, I think I have. I don't know how to love my body," I said. "But it's clear that right now, I have to learn."

This revelation was followed by a sudden horrible fear: Is it too late to learn to love myself? Is it too late to heal my wounded body?

After I left Will's office, I went to the natural-foods store in Providence and bought some staples, and then went home. I was no sooner in my kitchen and putting my groceries down when the telephone rang. A woman who introduced herself as Sun Kim was answering my newspaper ad requesting help with Oriental-style cooking. Sun said she was Korean and could help me with Asian-food preparation. As it turned out, hers was the only answer I would receive.

Later that week Sun arrived at my house at about 9 A.M., and together we went through the macrobiotic cookbooks to determine if she knew the foods I needed help preparing.

I pointed to a page at random. "Miso? Do you know what miso is?" I asked.

"Ah, yes," she said. "My mother made miso at home."

"Good, good," I said. "Do you know how to make miso soup?"

"Yes, I know," she said.

"Brown rice. Do you know how to pressure-cook brown rice?" I asked.

"Yes, I can pressure-cook. Normally, we eat white rice in Korea, but we can make brown rice if you like," she said.

"Wonderful," I said.

I liked Sun instantly. Only in her early thirties, she was petite, delicate, and beautiful, with large dark eyes, short black hair, and a small mouth that seemed always to be turning into a smile or a laugh. Sun's husband was a graduate student at Brown University, where he was studying for a PhD in mathematics. They had two boys, six and eight years old, both of whom attended a local grammar school. That left time for Sun to come to my house twice a week to help me prepare a few days' worth of meals.

About half the foods in the macrobiotic books were familiar to Sun. The other half, we'd learn together. So began our mutual adventure in macrobiotic cooking. Every Monday and Wednesday, Sun came to my house and together we cooked for several hours. Sun, it turned out, was a much better cook than I. She had a certain artistic flair with the food and liked to make the dishes look—as well as taste—good. She knew how to use many of the Japanese foods, such as miso and tamari—the latter being a fermented soybean liquid—as bases for soups, stews, and noodle broths.

There were numerous foods that neither of us knew how to prepare, like *hijiki* seaweed, bulgur wheat, and burdock root. Sun didn't have a clue what to do with tempeh, a fermented soybean patty. *Seitan,* the gluten from wheat that has a meaty consistency and is frequently used as a meat substitute in vegetarian cooking, was a mystery to both of us. In such times we muddled through, experimenting with the amount of water or salt the dish might need, how much tamari or shoyu to use, what vegetables we might combine, and how long a food should be cooked.

We learned to make miso soup so that the miso and vegetables drowned out the flavor of the seaweed. We made *udon* noodles in tamari broth, with shiitake mushrooms, leeks, and some thinly sliced collard greens or broccoli. The *udon* noodles—thick, traditional-style Japanese noodles made of sifted wheat—were delicious in the slightly salty tamari-vegetable broth. Sometimes we added tempeh to the broth to make it rich and hearty. We learned how to use *mochi*—pounded sweet rice that was highly glutinous—in soup. When boiled in soup, the *mochi* became plump, like dumplings. Some of the *mochi* would break off from the larger dumplings, filling the soup broth to make it hearty and rich. Sometimes I combined *miso* broth with mochi and watercress, a rich and delicious meal in itself that I came to love. We used lots of exotic foods, such as *fu,* a wheat gluten that was rolled up and used in soup; lotus root, a vegetable with holes in it that macrobiotic practitioners maintained was good for the lungs; and *natto,* fermented soybeans that I initially found very odd-tasting but later came to enjoy as a condiment on rice or in noodles. We boiled bulgur wheat and added sauerkraut to make it tasty. We learned how to make healthful sauces using tofu, miso, or rice vinegar. We made pickles in miso or salt. We made all kinds of vegetable medleys, sometimes adding sliced pieces of *seitan* for added flavor. We also used *seitan* in stews and noodle broths. And we learned how to pressure-cook brown rice until it tasted nutty and sweet, especially when chewed consistently.

In the course of all this cooking, Sun and I became a good team. Sun's nature matched her name. She seemed to take pleasure in everything we did together, even when a dish completely bombed. And that happened on a fairly regular basis. Still, most dishes came out remarkably well, and it wasn't long before I actually started to enjoy most of the macrobiotic foods.

Meanwhile, we shared our respective struggles with life. Sun told me about her life in Korea, how poor her family was, and that her family's best hope of escaping poverty was for Sun and her husband to come to America. The golden thread that led to success in America was education, Sun and her husband said. They stressed it for themselves and especially for their children. Though they were highly ambitious, the Kim family was friendly, open, and eager to learn American ways. For Sun and her family, America was their one great chance at a new life. In a strange way, I saw Sun in similar terms. She made macrobiotics possible for me.

She also freed me considerably to make standard American fare for my children. With the exception of my oldest son, Sean, who was more accepting, they had rejected macrobiotics completely. Most of the foods were tasteless, they said, and those that they could taste were impossible to swallow. They were constantly making jokes about the diet, which only served to reinforce their rejection of the diet. Initially, I rejected their reaction entirely. "No," I said. "You can't have milk or sugary foods anymore. We're eating macrobiotically from now on."

What a fight ensued! "No way, Mom," my son Damian cried. "I can't eat that stuff. I'm going on strike," he said. My other children were equally resistant. Part of their resistance came from the fact that they didn't know how perilous my situation was, nor how dependent I was on the macrobiotic diet to heal myself.

A conversation I had with my oldest son, Christopher, who was seventeen at the time, clarified a lot for me.

"Mom, why are you eating these strange foods?" he asked me just after I began macrobiotics.

"I'm using this food to help my health," I said. "As you know, I haven't been well for a long time, and I think this diet will help me."

"We want you to get better, Mom, but we can't eat this way. We're not sick and we don't like the taste of this food."

"Okay," I said. "I understand. I'll cook the same way I used to for you kids, okay?"

From that day forward, I cooked two sets of meals every night—one for me and Keven, and one for my children. Keven would eat from both sides of the street, so to speak, but mostly he ate the macrobiotic foods.

Preparing two sets of meals every night was extremely difficult. In fact, it was possible only because I had Sun helping me prepare macrobiotic meals during the week. In addition to Sun, Eileen Shea occasionally came to my house to cook meals, or I would pick up meals-to-go from her house. If it were not for these two women, macrobiotics would not have been possible for me, I believe.

In a very short time I got to know Eileen and came to better understand her dedication to macrobiotics. As with many people who practiced this way of life, Eileen's dedication was rooted in gratitude.

In 1976 Eileen was living in Boca Raton, Florida, still in her mid-twenties and the mother of a four-year-old son. Her son was suffering from chronic ear infections. After numerous specialists, an endless number of tests, and just as many drugs, her son's condition remained unchanged. One day a friend told her that a Japanese man by the name of Michio Kushi was coming to Boca Raton to lecture on macrobiotics, a diet and lifestyle that was reputed to improve health. The word macrobiotics meant nothing to Eileen, but she decided to go on the off-chance that she might talk to Mr. Kushi about her son's ear infections.

"I was skeptical, but the lecture he gave was very interesting," Eileen recalled many years later. "After he finished his talk, I went to the front of the auditorium, stood in line to meet him, and when I finally got my chance, I asked him about my son's ear infections. He looked at my little boy and then said that my son's problems came from dairy food and sugar. I had stopped eating meat some time before, but I was eating tons of dairy food and still some sugar. So was my son. But then Mr. Kushi turned to me and said, 'If you and your son stop dairy food, you'll both get better and your reproductive problems will clear up.' That floored me. I hadn't said a word about any reproductive problems, but in fact I had had a large ovarian cyst removed three years before and I was having trouble getting pregnant at the time.

"'How do you know that I have reproductive problems?' I asked him.

"'Please study and you'll learn and share it with other people,' he said.

"There were other people waiting to talk to him, so I thanked him and left, but after that I began to study macrobiotics very carefully. At first, I didn't love the macrobiotic food and I hated seaweed. I didn't know how to cook, so I went to Boston and studied cooking with Aveline Kushi, Michio's wife, and other macrobiotic teachers. Pretty soon, I became very careful with my diet. Some people thought I was fanatical, but my reproductive problems cleared up and I had three more children."

While she was studying macrobiotics, Eileen's twin sister, Elaine, suffered a deep depression. Eileen urged her sister to adopt the macrobiotic diet, which Eileen believed could help her overcome her depression. Elaine was living in Massachusetts at the time, not far from Newburyport, where a macrobiotic-cooking teacher by the name of Patricia Murray ran a kind of macrobiotic bed-and-breakfast. Elaine stayed with Pat Murray for a while, studied cooking, ate the food, and in a short time overcame her depression.

In the meantime, Eileen's elderly aunt developed breast cancer. Eileen got a macrobiotic counselor to visit her aunt in the hospital. Eileen and Elaine made food for their aunt and placed her on a strict macrobiotic diet.

"My aunt ended up dying, but I saw her improve several times and she lived longer than anyone expected," Eileen said. "The quality of her life was so much better than if she had just done chemotherapy or radiation. That was another sign to me of just how powerful macrobiotics could be."

In 1982, the two sisters opened the East West Center in Providence, initially out of Eileen's home. Eventually, they moved to DePasquale Square and their cozy little storefront.

"Before we opened up the center, I used to shop at the local natural-foods store, Golden Sheaf," Eileen recalled. "The guy who owned the store didn't have many macrobiotic staples, so I asked him to order them. The more he ordered, the more he sold. One day he told me that his business had doubled since he began stocking macrobiotic foods. I was amazed. Apparently a macrobiotic community was springing up in the greater Providence area. When Michio Kushi's son, Phiya, asked me if I would start an East West Center in Providence, it seemed perfect. I wanted to help people and this seemed like a really good way to do it."

I was now another of those people Eileen was helping, and I couldn't have been more grateful. Keven and I attended macrobiotic dinners every Friday night at the East West Center. In the first few weeks after our first dinner at the center, the only activity was a dinner for the community. People gathered and talked mostly about their experiences with macrobiotics. Many went to Boston, where Michio Kushi and other macrobiotic teachers gave lectures. Whenever people returned from such events, they would share what they learned with the group. At such times people would gather around and listen to the person recount what Michio or some other teacher had talked about. Michio's lectures, we were told, usually combined both the practical and the philosophical aspects of macrobiotics, ranging from the use of food as a healing tool, to food's effects on mental and spiritual health. Keven particularly loved such discussions.

As he said many times, the dinners at the East West Center reminded him of the community cells of the civil rights movement during the 1960s. People were galvanized by the ideas that Michio and others were presenting. Not only were they talking about physical health, but also about the effects of health and illness on society and the world at large. Kushi maintained that not only could individual sickness be healed through macrobiotics, but many social ills, as well. Violence and mental disorders could be drastically reduced if people changed their ways of eating. The use of yin and yang as a tool for understanding human health, thinking, and behavior took macrobiotics into another realm, beyond individual health, to world peace.

Remarkably, the macrobiotic philosophy went even further. By eating grains and vegetables, Kushi maintained, people would gain a greater sensitivity for the feelings and needs of others and for spirit itself. Once, as we drove home from a Friday night gathering, Keven said that these ideas, coupled with the air of reverence toward the food and the fact that so many people were using the food to heal themselves of disease, gave macrobiotics a kind of spiritual feeling that he dearly appreciated. Without being a religion, macrobiotics presented ideas that form the basis for a certain philosophical and spiritual way of life.

Just as much as he loved the ideas and the Friday night gatherings, Keven enjoyed the food, especially the food prepared by Eileen and Elaine. Even the seaweed seemed fine with him. A whole new side of my husband seemed to be emerging before my eyes. He was temperamentally suited to a vegetarian diet, even though he had spent his entire adult life as a lawyer and a politician, two professions one hardly associates with vegetarianism and spirituality. Yet, there he was, deeply engaged in these Friday night talks, which ranged from food and health to humankind's ultimate diet.

For my part, I saw the macrobiotic diet as my chance at survival, at least that was my initial view. I remained absolutely strict to the letter of the law. Health is taken for granted when you're healthy, but when you're ill, health is the most precious commodity on earth. I wanted my health back and I was willing to adhere strictly to Marc Van Cauwenberg's original dietary recommendations. I didn't dare deviate a whit.

Right from the start the food had a strange effect on me. The meals in general left me feeling full—with all those vegetables, there was lots of fiber and bulk—but also light. I never got up from the table feeling stuffed or bloated. On the contrary, the macrobiotic foods made me feel lighter, as if my organs weren't as strained as they had been on my old diet.

The foods that had the most immediate effect on me were miso soup, which always made me hungry, but at the same time slightly stronger and clearer of mind, and brown rice. Brown rice was the staple grain, though other grains, such as barley, millet, oats, and wheat were used frequently, as well. Whole, unprocessed grains gave me a distinct sense of well-being. There was no mistaking the feeling after a bowl of rice: I felt a little more stable, a little more balanced, and a lot more energetic. I knew this because I was usually weak. I also had the feeling of being emotionally and physically brittle, as if my nervous system was tingling and irritated at the surface of my skin. After a bowl of grain, this brittle feeling subsided. In its place was a sense of relaxation and calm. I would later learn that grain boosts serotonin, a chemical neurotransmitter that the brain uses to create feelings of well-being and enhanced concentration. But long before I had such information, I realized that whole grains made me feel more integrated and strangely in harmony with my surroundings, what people often refer to as being "centered." Rice and other grains also gave me the feeling of being full and sated. For this reason, grains were considered the center of the meal, much as meat is considered the center of most modern American meals.

Other foods had a palpable effect, as well. Leafy greens, such as collards, kale, and mustard greens, were extremely chewy and fibrous, but if I ate a meal dominated by these foods, I felt a gnawing sensation in my stomach—even my whole body—as if my body were attempting to draw food and sustenance to itself. Clearly, I could not live on green vegetables alone. Squash, such as acorn, butternut, buttercup, and *Hokkaido* pumpkin, filled me up.

All these fibrous foods had a tremendous effect on my digestion and elimination. After suffering from chronic constipation for many years, I now had the opposite problem. It seemed that nothing stayed inside me very long. I called Marc Van Cauwenberg and complained that I had frequent bowel movements and sometimes diarrhea. He told me to eat *natto* beans once a day for a couple of weeks. Marc said I should cook the *natto* beans for a few minutes in a little miso and chopped scallions. *Natto* beans are fermented soybeans. Fermentation provides friendly bacteria that would help my digestion, Marc said. The beans have a very sticky and stringy consistency and an odd taste and smell that takes most people some time to get used to.

When I cooked the beans the first time, a very pungent, almost acrid odor filled the house. Mary Kathryn and Damian came running into the kitchen, holding their noses. "What is that awful smell," they cried out. Then Damian ran out of the house, yelling, "I'm not coming back until that smell is gone!"

The *natto* beans, as far as my children were concerned, were just another good reason to reject macrobiotics.

Remarkably, the cooked *natto* beans did strengthen my digestion and stopped the diarrhea.

All of these foods combined to create the most demanding set of cravings I had ever encountered. I craved sugar as if it were a drug, and I was addicted. In fact, I really was addicted to sugar, I realized. Before I began the macrobiotic diet, I ate chocolate, usually fudge, every night before I went to bed. I kept jelly beans and caramels on my desk and ate them throughout the day. I drank several sodas daily and never retreated from desserts. In other words, I ate sugar all day long.

Now, after my encounter with Marc Van Cauwenberg, I dared not go near the stuff. He made it clear that my very life depended on my avoiding sugar entirely. It was one of the toughest things I have ever done. Only hours after I stopped eating it, my entire body seemed to scream out for chocolate. And that scream only got louder before it started to come under control. The withdrawal symptoms from my addiction were wretched. I broke out in cold sweats and suffered severe headaches. I got anxiety. My hands shook. I had terrible attacks of hypoglycemia, or low blood sugar, which brought about sudden periods of fatigue, weakness, and irritability. The craving for sugar was acute whenever I started feeling weak, tired, and depressed.

To combat these intense cravings, Marc had instructed me to eat a sweet vegetable, such as cooked squash, carrots, or parsnips. If these foods weren't available, eat a bowl of rice or any vegetables that were available, he said. Yet, nothing satisfied the craving entirely and it wouldn't be long before I was craving the stuff again. The best I could do to stave off the cravings was fill up on grains and vegetables, which would give me an hour or so before the cravings rose again. But even after a meal, I craved some sweet dessert—anything. Instead, I drank my *bancha* twig tea. The tea settled me somewhat and took the edge off the cravings for a while, but they were never far from my consciousness.

And then came the discharges. Marc Van Cauwenberg and others had warned me that my cancer was triggered and supported by toxins that had accumulated in my tissues over many years. In fact, Marc had said that the tumors my body was producing were themselves forms of discharge. My body was expelling the toxins that supported and fostered the cancer inside me. In order to overcome my cancer, I had to eliminate those toxins that were now supporting its growth. The poisons he was referring to were essentially sugar, fat, cholesterol, and artificial colors, flavors, pesticides, and other ingredients that filled my fat cells. Once I went on the macrobiotic diet, my body would start to eliminate these poisons, Marc had said. He called this process of purging the toxins "discharging."

Pretty soon I was discharging like crazy. I had bumps and rashes and pimples coming out of my skin like you wouldn't believe.

Some of those skin eruptions were tumors that I continued to produce all over my body. These appeared either as scablike projections that emerged on the upper part of my back and chest, or as hardened pimples that were probably lymph nodes that had become swollen and solid.

And then I started to lose weight. Since my operation in March, I weighed barely ninety-five pounds. But after about two weeks on the macrobiotic diet, it was clear that I was losing more weight, and fast. As with the discharges, Marc had warned me that I would lose a few pounds. The weight loss would also facilitate the elimination of toxins that had accumulated around my organs and inside my tissues, he said. He also assured me that the weight would come back. But between the weight loss and skin discharges, I began to look even sicker. My appearance terrified me. All I had to do was to look in the mirror to know my cancer was now rampaging through my body. I lapsed into moments of absolute terror.

Those around me were understandably afraid, as well. People would say, "Marlene, you've got to eat meat, eggs, and milk products to keep your strength up. You look terrible and you're losing weight. That diet is killing you." Frankly, I didn't know what to answer.

Fortunately, Al came to our house frequently and reassured me that my body was just cleansing itself as part of the healing process. "Marc said that these would be signs that you are getting better, Marlene," Al would remind me.

One day toward the end of May, I telephoned Marc in a panic and confessed that the weight loss worried me immensely.

"How are you feeling?" Marc asked. "How is your energy level?"

"I feel about the same, Marc," I said. "I actually think I've got a little more energy than I did before I saw you."

"What are your latest blood-test results?" he asked.

I had been having monthly blood tests even after the surgery at Mass General. I went over some of the test results with Marc, but the one he seemed most concerned about was my hematocrit, which had remained below normal, even after the surgery.

"How is your appetite? Do you get hungry?" Marc asked.

"Yes, I'm hungry all the time," I said. "And I'm craving sugar constantly."

"Don't worry about the weight loss," Marc said. "You will lose a little weight and then your weight will stabilize. In a few months you may even gain a few pounds back. Just be patient. The most important thing is that your appetite is good and your energy is improving. As soon as you have discharged more of the sugar, you'll stop craving it so much. I think you're doing fine for the time being."

One thing I did notice that suggested improved health was that my blood was bright red now. In the past, it was always dark brown. I noticed one day when I got my menstrual cycle that my blood had changed dramatically from its previous dark color to a bright red. What had happened, I wondered.

Marc assured me that this was another good sign and that my body would now begin healing. The redness, he said, was a sign that my blood contained more hemoglobin and more oxygen. It also contained fewer toxins, the very substances that were supporting the growth of the cancer, Marc said.

Whenever I talked to Marc, which I did every few weeks, I felt reassured. But such reassurance would be short-lived. Nighttime was often the worst part of the day. It was almost as if death were a little closer at night. Invariably, some kind of pain would arise and I would envision malignant cells spreading throughout my small intestine.

Often the fear overwhelmed me. One night, while we lay in bed, I began to hyperventilate. "I think I'm dying, Keven. I think the cancer is spreading inside of me right now. I can almost feel it." I shook uncontrollably.

"Breathe, Marlene," Keven said. "It's going to be all right. You're fine. Really. Take deep breaths." Marc had instructed me to breathe deeply and rhythmically to help bring the fear under greater control.

But I couldn't. "I don't want to leave the children, I don't want to leave you! I don't want to die."

"Marlene, you're not going to die," Keven said. "You're going to make it. Breathe, please. Exhale. Let it out."

I had to get out of bed and walk around. I paced the room, trying to get hold of my breath. I tried as best I could to take long breaths, but as soon as I started to get a little control, the fear would rise inside of me and I'd be panicking and hyperventilating again.

"Let's pray," Keven said. "Let's ask God for help."

We said the Lord's Prayer together out loud and then we said about ten Hail Marys. The prayer to the Holy Mother soothed and calmed me. I started breathing more rhythmically. I was coming down from the terrifying heights. I was exhausted.

"I believe macrobiotics is going to work, Marlene," Keven said. "This isn't just another alternative cancer treatment. There's something here, I believe. There's really something of substance and truth here. Besides, what choice did we have?

There was nothing in medicine that was going to help you. We looked. We heard what they were offering. This is the best that life presented to us. I know it's going to get us through this thing. You know what? I think it's helping you already, Marlene. I really believe that."

"Do you think so, Keven?" I asked.

"Yes. I really do. The signs are small but we've got to give it time. I think you'd be a lot worse today if you weren't following the diet. I really believe that. You've got to continue to be strict and careful, just like you have been. Why don't you call Marc or Eileen tomorrow?"

The thought of talking to Marc or Eileen made me feel better. They always seemed to know what to say to me.

Though I did not immediately have any proof that macrobiotics was improving my health, it gave me hope. Right from the start, macrobiotics offered me a set of tools that I could use to overcome my cancer. The diet was a daily practice, a practical set of behaviors that I could do for myself. It gave me a certain amount of power and independence. I didn't have to surrender to doctors. More important, I didn't take chemotherapy, which most certainly would have debilitated my body and perhaps broken my spirit. Instead I had the macrobiotic belief, which I was trying to internalize, that the diet and lifestyle would strengthen my body's healing mechanisms, which were sufficient to overcome cancer.

Keven was right, I thought. There were no other choices being offered to me. This was my path.

CHAPTER 6

Return to Spiritual Life

The Friday night dinners at the East West Center had become a ritual for Keven and me. It wasn't long before we knew almost everyone who came each week, and increasingly, there was a sense of shared purpose and community. Coming to the East West Center reminded me that I was not alone.

It also reminded me of what the source of all healing was. After the meal was served and we sat down at the table, everyone paused to say a silent prayer of thanksgiving. On the surface, it seemed like such a little thing, but the redirection of our attention away from the social event to the divine changed the atmosphere of the room and the attitudes of the people in it. We were suddenly reverent—not reverent of the food, but the Source that provided it. The food was the Creator's gift. We acknowledged the connection and thus understood the source of its healing power.

Eating in this manner was itself a prayer. This silent thanksgiving put everything in perspective for me. In that small moment my life seemed properly aligned, my priorities in order. It was a moment of peace, gratitude, and understanding.

In this way, macrobiotics was changing my life fundamentally. It wasn't just the food that was changing me, but the *values* of macrobiotics were affecting me so deeply and were changing my outlook. Macrobiotics, I realized, was more than just a diet, but a spiritual way of living. Just as Michio Kushi had written, macrobiotics was making me more spiritually aware.

Interestingly, that spiritual awareness had almost nothing to do with religion. I was a practicing Roman Catholic, but there were Buddhists, Protestants, Jews, and even an Arab or two among us. It didn't matter what our backgrounds might be. Nothing in macrobiotics contradicted any of the major religious traditions, at least as far as I could see. If anything, it supported every religious expression, perhaps because the practice rested on universal values, such as our common need for health and the power of food to enhance or destroy health.

Following Marc Van Cauwenberg's instructions, I chewed my food thoroughly, at least thirty-five to fifty times a mouthful. I noticed that the more I chewed, the tastier the food became. This was especially true of grain. I was learning that grain started out tasting bland, but after it was chewed for a time, it released its sugars and was suddenly sweet and very satisfying. I realized that the more I chewed, the better I liked the food. Unfortunately, that experience did not extend to seaweed, which I continued to detest. Usually I mixed it with another vegetable on my plate or just ate it as I would a foul-tasting medicine. I had read that seaweed was rich in nutrients—especially in beta-carotene and minerals—which were essential for my healing. But knowing a food was good for me did not make it palatable. Still, the grains and vegetables were definitely growing on me.

There was only sporadic conversation during the meal, as most people ate in silence. When the meal was completed, however, the conversation rose again. Someone had a new recipe to share or a suggestion on how to make a particular dish tastier. Our discussions ranged far and wide, including all that was important to us—our jobs, our children, the daily problems that life presented. Even such mundane matters were viewed through the lens of macrobiotics. Someone at our table might start talking about their aggressive or dominating boss, and immediately someone else would observe, "Oh, he's too yang. He needs more yin—lots of vegetables and fruit. Or maybe a warm bath."

"I'd like to drown him in a warm bath," our friend said.

Inevitably people at our table would ask me how I was doing with the diet. At first, I was apprehensive about recognizing what I perceived to be small changes. I was afraid of indulging in false hope. Yet, I clearly felt more energetic, lighter, and clearer of mind. I still got tired; my energy rose and fell in waves, but when it was up, I perceived it to be stronger than it had been before I began macrobiotics.

There were other changes, just as subtle, that I was beginning to perceive. Up until the time I adopted the diet, I looked like death. Large hollows marked my sallow cheeks. My eyes literally drooped with exhaustion, as if announcing that my spirit had surrendered. The life energy in my body was leaving, that much was clear.

Marc Van Cauwenberg had said that I was *sanpaku*, a Japanese term that connotes "three whites showing." It meant that the sclera below the pupil of the eye was showing, along with the sclera to the left and right of the pupil. Only the sclera to the left and right of the pupil should be showing, according to the Japanese. Traditionally, *sanpaku* was seen as a sign that death was approaching. I shuddered to look in the mirror. Lately, however, I had begun to see faint changes in my face and eyes. My color was a little better, it seemed to me. But more important was that my eyes radiated more . . . well, life. My eyes seemed to emanate with a little more energy and strength. I attributed this largely to the improvement in my overall vitality. But the signs, though very small, reassured me. Could the diet be working? I could only pray that it was so.

Despite these small signs of progress, my doctors believed my condition was essentially unchanged. My blood tests consistently revealed the presence of disease. My hemoglobin tests, which indicated the number and health of my oxygen-carrying red blood cells, had been consistently below normal during the months leading up to my surgery in March, when my doctors discovered my cancer and then removed twenty-two inches of my small intestine. My hemoglobin had remained low, and my hematocrit levels were below normal. Even worse, my internist had discovered small amounts of blood in my stools and rectum. My doctors suggested that this was likely the result of the spreading cancer throughout my small and large intestines. As the cancer spread, it invaded blood vessels and released blood into the stools. This might explain why my hematocrit levels were so low.

The discovery of blood in my stools frightened me tremendously, because it was a sign that my cancer was still very much a part of me and still very active. There were other signs of disease, as well. I was still showing tiny tumors in my upper body, especially on my back and chest. In addition to these symptoms were a host of others that were equally frightening for a cancer patient, including skin rashes and headaches.

These "discharges" were a frequent subject at our Friday night dinners. It was commonly understood that the macrobiotic diet cleansed the system of all the old waste products and poisons that supported disease, including cancer, and that these toxins were often eliminated through the skin or as headaches and other discomforts. Such discharges, macrobiotic people maintained, were a sign of healing.

Everyone had their own discharge stories. Some were truly bizarre, such as the man, also with cancer, whose tongue turned black for a few months. When he went to Michio

Kushi for a consultation, Michio told him that his liver was cleansing itself and that the color of his tongue would return to normal—as long as he continued to eat well. In fact, his tongue did return to normal. Many people had had odd forms of elimination through the skin. One woman I met had a large bump appear on the left side of her back. The thing became as large as a plum and turned green.

"I was told by a macrobiotic counselor to apply a taro root plaster over the bump," she told me. Taro root is a small potatolike vegetable. To make a plaster using taro root, people grated it onto cheesecloth and then put a couple of drops of tamari into the grated taro root. The plaster draws toxins out of the skin and tissues below. "I taped the plaster onto my back, over the bump," the woman said, "and slept with the plaster on. One night the thing burst open as I was asleep and drained the entire night. When I woke up and removed the plaster, there was a clean, open wound there. The cheesecloth had absorbed the fluids. From that point on, I've had a scar there—it looks like a gash in my back."

Perhaps the most common form of elimination and cleansing, at least from the macrobiotic point of view, were colds and flus. Macrobiotics held that the common cold is good for you and even a sign of the body's inherent strength. A cold is the body's attempt to cleanse its system and to force the person with the cold to rest. Sneezing, runny nose, frequent urination, and diarrhea are the body's efforts to expel toxins that have accumulated within the system. Fever is the body's way of turning up the internal temperature and thereby creating internal conditions that kill the invading pathogen, such as a bacteria or virus. The typical symptoms of a cold or flu are therefore the outward signs that the body is cleansing itself and ridding itself of the underlying causes of disease. Even cancer cells—as well as the substances that support cancer—could be eliminated through the skin, mucus membranes, bowels, or urine. Medications only served to suppress the symptoms and therefore block the body's efforts at ridding itself of illness. In the long run, this only weakens the body's house-cleansing functions, its immune system.

Underlying this philosophy was the basic belief that the body can and does heal itself—at least when given the right conditions. Those "right conditions" were the macrobiotic way of life.

"Ohsawa said we should be grateful for sickness," someone said to me during one of these Friday dinners. The person was quoting George Ohsawa, the Japanese philosopher who had combined and developed the teachings of several ancient and traditional cultures, especially those of China, Japan, and Europe. He combined and integrated these teachings and called his philosophy macrobiotics, or "large life" or "great life." Ohsawa stressed the importance of gratitude so much that he made it a condition of health. If you weren't grateful for everything that came to you—the good and the bad—you had no chance of being truly healthy. Gratitude, said Ohsawa, was the basis of love. A person who loved only the good things in life, the rewards, was incapable of love that endured. He or she could never love through "thick and thin," through good times and bad, because the minute things became difficult, his love would evaporate. On the other hand, the person who is grateful for everything, including sickness and difficulties, is capable of truly loving life fully, because life is made up of both yin and yang, light and dark, happiness and sadness. Such a person could be happy and truly healthy.

Such conversations not only enlightened but inspired me. Yet, no matter what we talked about at these dinners, there was a sense of peace and even of spirit in the room. The room had atmosphere, though I was reluctant to say why, even to myself. Certainly, it was small and intimate. Moreover, people talked openly about very serious issues, including life and death, and I gradually found it possible to do likewise. Unlike so much of my past behavior, which might be best characterized as running away from myself, I was now forced to confront my life directly. I could no longer deny the complaints of my body or my heart. I had to learn to nurture myself and even to love myself in a whole new way. Macrobiotics forced me to become more introspective and more sensitive to my needs.

There was a lightness and a playfulness in the air, as well, for the people had great faith in the macrobiotic approach. Most of the people there truly believed that this diet and lifestyle could reverse their illnesses and restore their lives. The fact that so many of the people in the room had had such experiences—Tom Marron and Eileen and Elaine, being just three examples—gave all of us hope. But there was more. There was also the sense of reunion with the spirit and the recognition that spirit was the source of healing. That reunion was facilitated by the prayer before the meal and the topics we talked about, which always seemed to concern the most important aspects of life. In any case, many people recognized a kind of spiritual transformation occurring in their lives, just as I did. For me, the natural reaction to such a feeling was to return to my religious roots, which was Roman Catholicism.

Going Home

Before I developed cancer, I was what you might call "a good churchgoer." I went to mass every Sunday, as well as on the religious holidays. I also went for reconciliation, what used to be called "confession" before Vatican II, and regularly took Communion on Sundays. I believed in the basic tenets of my religion and tried to lead a religious life, as best as I understood it then. Indeed, from all outward appearances, I was a religious person. But now I realized that though I observed the letter of the law, I did not understand its spirit. It was one thing to be religious, but another to be spiritual. That distinction had been creeping up on me since I was diagnosed with cancer, and it was becoming more clear with my practice of macrobiotics.

Up until the time I got cancer, I was too busy to be spiritual. I didn't realize it, of course; as I said, I thought of myself as a spiritual person. But my spiritual life had been taken from me, ever so slowly and subtly, without my even realizing that it was gone. It happened over many years and, ironically, I participated in its loss. The principal means by which I lost my spiritual life were fear, external demands, and speed. Fear always made me hurry more. And the more stress or fear I had in my life, the faster I ran. My focus narrowed. All I could see was the goal or the chore that had to be accomplished, which would get me out of trouble.

The demands of my life arose partly out of my ambition for success, certainly, but my ambition was not the primary problem. I believed that without certain accomplishments—professional success, financial security, and a good family life—I could not feel good about myself, nor could I feel safe. My own self-worth and safety rested with what I had or had not attained.

I had never really felt safe since my father died. I decided early in life that I had to be the one to provide for myself. And so I drove myself relentlessly to achieve success, which to my mind meant security and safety. The surprise was that chasing success and security only brought more insecurity into my life. The more I did to be successful, the more demands I attracted into my life. And the more demands I faced, the more, things could go wrong for me. My life teetered precariously on the outcomes of a thousand appointments. Pretty soon, every new deal seemed like a life-and-death issue. At times it seemed that I was stretched across the entire state of Rhode Island. Running to this appointment, hurrying to that one. *Go faster, Marlene, or die.* That was the mindset that was at the heart of all my problems. Go faster, or you'll lose clients, lose accounts, lose money, lose position, lose security, lose your possessions, lose your life. In some recess of my mind lived an eleven-year-old-girl who had just lost her father and was now terrified of all that might go wrong for her and her family. That little girl's fears coalesced into a dark chasm, a virtual black hole, which was death itself. I feared that if I did not protect myself, I would die, like my father. I would be next.

I had become an overachieving doer, a person driven by her own will. In a very real sense, I had lost my feminine nature. That is to say, I had lost that part of me that was receptive, passive, open, soft, and self-nurturing. I was cut off from my feelings, especially from the pain I suffered from having to neglect my needs. I had to suppress my need for love, for rest, for tenderness, for the experience of simply *being*. In the process I had lost all sense of harmony with my inner life and with nature.

My profession saw the feminine as weakness, of course. The world of finance is an old boy's club, and in order to fit in, you had to be as tough as the boys. In virtually every area of my life, the masculine dominated the feminine. I saw how important balance was to restoring sanity to my life. I saw, as well, how important balance was to my healing.

But balance is more than scheduling your life a little better. It is an intimate awareness of your physical, emotional, and psychological needs, and then being able to meet those needs. And then I realized that coming home to myself was really a return to my own spirit and spiritual life. An old Indian aphorism holds that no one approaches God as anything but a woman. In other words, when confronting the divine, we must be open, passive, and accepting of inspiration and direction. Only by being open and accepting could I receive inspiration from above. I needed to be guided now. I couldn't find the way on my own. When left to my own devices, I ran directly into hell. I was ready to be led.

In order to better listen to my own inner voice, I began to spend more time sitting quietly in church when there were no services going on. I would go into the church well after morning mass had concluded, or in the afternoons, when only a few people—most of them older women—would appear to light a candle and pray. The silence and serenity of the church during these hours was healing of itself. During the middle hours of the day, between late morning and late afternoon, the church was at its most beautiful for me. The afternoon light brightened the blue and red mosaics within the stained-glass windows. On the whole, the church was only dimly lit, but here and there, shafts of white light would come streaming in through an open window. The ceiling soared fifty feet or more above my head, and the center aisle to the altar seemed like a long journey for the soul. The altar itself was the most brightly lit place within the church. The silence in this magnificent place was palpable and soothing. It was almost as if the silence itself was alive. There was a presence here, and silence was its voice. The life that permeated this church crept inside my soul and stroked me as though I was a little child. I would pray fervently. Sometimes, unexpectedly, I would start to weep from sadness. Eventually my sadness would melt into compassion for myself and others and then, just as unexpectedly, I would feel gratitude. There were times when I felt the presence of God more in this silence than I did during the mass.

The church was not my only haven. Only a half hour from my home is the shrine of La Salette in Attleboro, Massachusetts. The shrine commemorated the appearance of the Blessed Mother in 1846 when she appeared to two children. It is a place devoted to the reconciliation between humans and God.

La Salette encompasses eighty acres of grassy land, most of it crisscrossed by walkways. There is an array of buildings clustered together, among them a chapel, a dormitory of sorts, where people can stay overnight, a gift shop, and a cafeteria. The shrine's beautiful statues are its main focus, however. Among the statues are depictions of the Twelve

Stations of the Cross, or the twelve key events that marked Jesus' journey to Calvary and the Crucifixion. In addition, there is a Pietà on a tall hill and, on another hill, a statue of the Holy Mother.

I would come to La Salette in the early mornings, when few people, if anyone, were around. Sometimes I would recite prayers at the Stations of the Cross and at other times I would walk up the hill to the statue of the Holy Mother and just sit before the tall statue and pray. That was an especially peaceful thing to do because the statue is up on a hill and surrounded by shrubbery. It's very intimate and private, especially in the mornings, and a wonderful place to meditate and be alone with myself.

The statue must have stood nine or ten feet in height, and because it stood on a small embankment, it rose perhaps twelve to fifteen feet above my head. Her arms were outstretched, as if gathering her children to her. I came here and felt her welcome and her embrace.

On one perfect spring morning, I went to La Salette after my children went to school. I sat down on a little stone wall directly opposite the statue and felt myself sink into the moment and this place. My body relaxed and I took in the harmony that was all around me. It didn't last long. Whenever I got in touch with myself, the first feeling that arose inside of me was fear for my life. Usually I distracted myself immediately by thinking of something else. If I was in the car, I'd turn on the radio. If I was at the office or at home, I would find something to do to take my attention away from my feelings. Now, for some unexplainable reason, I just sat with my fear and felt it. At first, scenarios of leaving my children and husband came into my mind. My terror rose, but as I stayed within myself and didn't turn away, I felt my fear turn into anger. I didn't want to die. I didn't want to leave my family. I wanted to fight this disease. Indeed, I was fighting it—valiantly, I thought. That thought, that I was struggling as best I could, suddenly turned my anger into sadness and compassion for myself. I was doing my best, just as I had always done my best. Yes, sometimes doing what I thought was best got me more into trouble, but what else could I have done? I was struggling with life, as everyone is. It wasn't my fault, any more than it is anyone's fault. Once I realized this, my heart opened to myself and to others. Expectations dissolved like shadows suddenly flooded with light. Compassion for myself and all I had been through in life flowed up from below my stomach and into my heart. As I felt my pain and weakness, as I became aware of my terrible vulnerability, I felt the presence of the Blessed Mother draw near me.

I looked up at the statue and thought, Oh, Mother, take me into your arms and hold me close to your heart. Protect me from the darkness that is this cancer. Let me be your little child.

Suddenly I saw myself as a little girl, perhaps at the age of three, sitting on the living room floor, playing with my toys. My mother and father sat nearby on the couch. I was so happy. I was happy, I realized, just being me. I was enough. I didn't have to do anything to be worthy of love—in fact, the question of worthiness didn't even exist for me. I was alive and in love with life. Most of all, I loved my father and mother. We were a closed circle of love. I lived in the center of that circle, blissfully in the center of love.

In my mind's eye, the image suddenly changed. I was fourteen, my brother Al, seven. We were in our kitchen at home, setting the table for dinner. Vincent, my older brother, is out; he has his own life. My mother suddenly arrives home from work. She enters the house and hurries into the kitchen. Al and I greet her. "Hi, Mom," says Al. "Hi, Mom," I say. "How was your day, Mom?"

"Fine," she says, oblivious to the question.

Our mother's face is tight and drawn. It carries all the tension of the day, as does her entire body. She is still moving at the speed of work, quickly, nervously, preoccupied with getting the job done. The job is dinner. She has no awareness of herself. She has no awareness of how much she is driving herself, nor how much she needs to be cared for. Doing is survival for my mother. It is the safe haven away from her feelings, away from her pain, away from the absence of my father. Al and I retreat from the kitchen to the living room. We sit down on the couch and I am aware of how much I want to be close to him, to protect him. The television is on. We're huddled on the couch, watching television, absorbed in our own world. The circle that once held me and my parents no longer exists. It has been broken and re-formed around Al and me. We are the circle of love now. In some basic and essential way, my mother is gone, lost to all her fears, her responsibility, her doing. This, I would realize much later, is the standard life pattern for single mothers.

As I sat before the statue of the Holy Mother, I realized how painfully in need I was of mothering. Holy Mother, I thought, be with me. I am your child. I am that little girl, still in need of mothering. Help me, help our family. I could not hold back the tears, but after crying a bit, the peace I had experienced when I first sat down to pray was back. I had come full circle. Only now, I felt purged of all the darkness that I was carrying when I came here that morning. It was as if a dam that held so much pain within me had suddenly given way, and my pent-up emotions flowed from me until the waters were clean and clear again.

From my pocket I took out a little slip of paper on which was printed a prayer to my old childhood friend, St. Jude, the patron saint of lost causes. I said the words as the tears rolled freely down my cheeks:

> *"Sacred heart of Jesus,*
> *pray for us.*
> *St. Jude worker of miracles,*
> *pray for us.*

St. Jude, help of the
the helpless, pray for us."

Truly, I felt as if I had come home again.

La Salette became a refuge. I went there often, especially
in the early mornings or evenings during the week, when I
could be alone. Only when the place was vacant could I really
feel its spirit, but what a wonderful spirit it was that permeated the grounds. Like a church when it is empty, La Salette
had its own characteristic energy that was unmistakable and
healing. There were many reports of people who had miracu-
lously overcome sickness or physical handicap after visiting
La Salette. The most important thing that happened to me
was that at La Salette, I reconnected to my inner spirit and to
the Holy Mother, which I came to believe was fundamental to
my healing. I would not get well by food alone, I now knew,
but by using food, prayer, and every other form of healing to
reconnect with my soul. The power to heal sprang from the
healing waters that flowed from a divine source. Now I
needed to find that source in everything I did.

The First Sign of Light

During the first week in July, Marc Van Cauwenberg came
to Rhode Island to teach and do personal consultations in a
local hotel room. As he had done when we first met, he gave
me a thorough examination. He looked carefully at my face
and then at the sclera of my eyes, asking me to look up so he
could examine the sclera below the iris; look down, to see
above the iris; left and right, so he could look at the sides. He
examined my arms, especially my forearms, and my feet. As
he conducted his examination, my heart pounded. What
signs of cancer was he looking for? What veins in my eyes,
what colors in my face, what telltale symptoms on my arms

and feet would give my condition away? My life seemed to hang on his breath. What did his barely audible "hmmm" mean? Was it life or death, Marc?

Once the examination was over, he resumed his seat behind his desk and smiled.

"You're making progress, Marlene. How do you feel?"

"I really think I'm starting to feel better," I answered. "I am more energetic. I sleep better and I wake up with more energy. I still get tired during the day, especially around three P.M., but around four or five I'm feeling my energy come back. I think I look better, too. I don't have that death mask I used to have," I said.

In fact, I had the strong impression that I looked significantly brighter and fuller in the face. The deep fatigue and anomie that were in my eyes were gradually being replaced by a palpable clarity and a level gaze. Was I less *sanpaku* now? I believed I was.

"I still have problems on the right side of my body, though," I told him. "I feel a little weaker on this side"—I pointed to my right arm—"and this is the side most of my tumors were on. Why do my problems all manifest on my right side?" I asked.

"For several reasons," he said, smiling. "First, your liver, which is on the right side of your body, is still very contracted and blocked, though far less so than it was when we first met. Your heart and small intestine meridians are also blocked. There's less life force circulating on your right side. In Chinese medicine, the heart and small intestine are related organs. One nourishes the other with *Qi*. Your cancer was found in your small intestine. The cancer arose there because the meridian was blocked and life force wasn't getting to the organ."

"Why was my small intestine so troubled?" I asked.

"First, your old way of eating, which was completely imbalanced, as I told you when we first met. Second, you have great difficulty taking care of yourself, or nourishing yourself.

The function of the small intestine is to take nutrition from our food and absorb it into our blood. Metaphorically, its purpose is to obtain what we need from life. You're a little weak in that area."

Marc's words hit home and brought other thoughts to the surface. I had read in one of the macrobiotic books that Oriental medicine associates the right side of the body with the mother and the left side with the father. I asked Marc about this and how it might relate to me. He thoughtfully explained in full detail.

"Oriental medicine is based on the idea that cosmic radiation is pouring down constantly on the earth and each of us from the sun, moon, and stars. Oriental medicine sees that radiation as 'heaven's force.' Meanwhile, the earth is spinning. If you plunge a ball into water and then spin the ball, droplets of water are flung off because centrifugal force drives the water away from the ball. The earth is doing the same thing: By spinning, it sends energy upward, away from the earth, as it turns on its axis. This creates a force that is radiating upward from below us. Earth's force is constantly showering us from below, while heaven's force rains down on us from above.

"In Chinese medicine and macrobiotics, heaven's force is seen as yang. It is associated with the male, or father, while earth's force is seen as yin and associated with the female, or mother. Even though heaven's force rains down on the entire body, it flows strongest on the left side, while earth's force flows most powerfully on the right side.

"Therefore, in Oriental diagnosis, our relationship with our father is seen on the left. Our relationship with our mother is seen on the right. Your problems are related to your ability to mother yourself. That means, to take care of and nurture yourself, as a mother would nurture you. You're not so good at that function yet.

"You might say that there is a certain relationship between mothering ourselves and recognizing what we need from life and being able to give it to ourselves, which metaphorically is related to the small intestine. So there is a kind of metaphorical and functional relationship between the small intestine and mothering energy."

Once again, my relationship with myself, my lifestyle, my body, and my mother were all tied together. I marveled that so many of my issues seemed tied up into a single package in my consciousness. I did not blame my mother in the least for my problems. On the contrary, I loved my mother. What I did feel bad about, however, was that I had known for years that my life was out of balance. Clearly, that was not my mother's fault. I was an adult. I was responsible for my own behavior and the way I cared for myself.

"Still, Marlene, let's focus on the positive," Marc said. "You're making progress, and frankly, it's greater progress than I had ever thought you would make. If anyone had asked me after our first meeting if you would adopt macrobiotics so religiously, I would have said, 'no.' You were the last person I thought would have adopted this way of life. Now let's make some adjustments in your diet."

Specifically, he decreased the amount of grain I ate and increased vegetables. He also asked me to do more lighter cooking. "Lightly steam your vegetables; cook them only a few minutes," he said. Marc explained that he was making these changes because it was springtime now and, like the season, I had to open up more and become more yin. More vegetables and lighter cooking would do that for me. "Grain should make up only forty percent of your meal. Make vegetables forty percent."

The rest of my diet, he said, should be beans, sea vegetables, soups, and condiments.

As we parted that day, Marc gave me a big, happy grin. Whenever he laughed, his whole body shook. "Keep up the good work, Marlene," he said. "You're doing wonderfully. I'll see you in August."

* * *

I left Marc as if I was walking on air. The diet was working. Something, finally, was working in my life.

My cancer had ravaged my body and brought me to the shore of death. Whatever small reserves I had left were stripped from me by my medical treatment, or so it seemed. I had been reduced to skin and bones, almost spiritless. When I originally saw Marc Van Cauwenberg, I was more cynical than even I realized. Deep down I had believed I was gone, my life was over. Every word that proffered some hope I cynically viewed as a sham. I had lost my faith.

But from all those dark embers had come a little light that—did I dare believe it?—now seemed to be a small, delicate flame. Was life being rekindled within? Could I hope? Yes, I could feel the desperate hope that rose with that tiny flame of health that was keeping me alive. I'm still alive, I told myself. I still have a chance.

CHAPTER 7

The Healing Power
of Surrender

After my consultation with Marc, something lifted inside me. I was palpably less afraid. I had begun to believe, perhaps even know in my bones, that I had turned a corner and was getting better. Once that belief settled, I stopped feeling so negative about my chances. I stopped thinking about death. Instead, I felt a joy and a sense of purpose. My progress reinforced my commitment to this practice and to the strictness with which I was following it.

My entire family seemed to know, if only intuitively, that some unexpressed darkness had lifted, as well. Occasionally, one or another of my children would come to the East West Center for Friday night dinners. I think they did it more out of curiosity than a desire to really know anything about macrobiotics. One night I brought Mary Kathryn to dinner. Everyone made a big fuss over her. I was proud as could be of her, as I was of all my children, especially at these dinners. I felt like a celebrity. All the people there knew I was making progress—I had shared my good news with several people after seeing Marc—and were telling Mary Kathryn how great I was. I couldn't imagine that she had any idea what they were talking about. Besides that, she was shy, and everything around her was strange and foreign.

Once we got our meals and sat at our table, Mary Kathryn noticed that everyone was using chopsticks. I had gotten her silverware, but next to her knife and fork was a pair of chopsticks. "What are these things, Mom?" she asked, holding up a pair.

"They're chopsticks, honey. People in Japan and China use them instead of forks and knives."

"That's strange," she said. She placed them in her hand and tried to manipulate them as best she could. "How do you do it?" she asked.

I fixed the two sticks in her hand and manipulated her fingers to make the sticks clamp together. I then held up a pair in my own hand and showed her how to do it, for by now, I felt like an old pro. She strained to make the sticks work and then tried to pick up a vegetable with them. She barley managed to get it off her plate before it fell back down.

"Good," I said. "You're getting it. But you know what? You've also got a fork and knife here, just in case you need them." I gave her a little wink and we both laughed.

From that day onward, Mary Kathryn regularly suggested that we go out to eat at a Japanese or Chinese restaurant so that she could try to eat with chopsticks again.

The spark of hope that had returned to my life also had a profound effect on my relationship with Keven. We were both more relaxed now and could talk about things other than my health. Also, I experienced fewer bouts of panic, which made him believe even more in my ability to get well. That is not to say that fear was gone, or that I did not have panic attacks anymore. On the contrary, I would still become inflamed with fear occasionally. When that happened, I would question Marc's assessment of my health. But those periods passed rather rapidly. The truth was, I trusted Marc and macrobiotics, and I clung to his assessment of my health as though it was life itself.

I wanted desperately to get away, if only for a weekend. My older brother, Vincent, arranged for us to have a condominium at Newport, Rhode Island, for two weeks. Keven and I immediately jumped at it. That was a blessing I will never forget—not because we did anything out of the ordinary. All we did was walk around town and on the beach. But the chance to be free of all the familiar surroundings was like being freed—if only on a furlough—from prison. One night Keven and I walked along the beach and then out on a jetty, where we looked out onto the horizon as the sun went down behind us. We held hands and talked about insignificant things. I looked at Keven and saw in his familiar face how much emotion and responsibility he was carrying on his shoulders. "God, we've been through a lot this year," I said. "My only hope is that next year, we're looking at each other in this same way." He patted my hand and smiled introspectively.

"I love you," I said.

"I love you, too."

None of my optimism, nor my sense of progress, was shared by my physicians. They were appalled by my practice of macrobiotics. At that time I was seeing three physicians: an oncologist, an internist, and a dermatologist. I was no longer seeing Dr. Cosimi, my surgeon, nor was I consulting my former dermatologist, Dr. Angermeier, who had left my HMO. My three current physicians were all new to me and all steadfastly against macrobiotics, which they regarded as charlatanism. My internist was the most adamantly opposed to macrobiotics, telling me at one point that I was likely doing myself harm. She even went so far as to sift through the medical archives for a critical article about macrobiotics that had been published years before in a medical journal.

"Here," she said. "I have something for you. It's an article about the diet you're on. I think after reading this you'll have second thoughts about what you are doing."

Frankly, I was appalled. One of the strands of hope from

which my life hung was macrobiotics. Indeed, it was one of my greatest sources of strength. I wondered whether this attempt to cut one of my lifelines was tantamount to a death wish. In any case, their attitude toward me was not unlike a kind of death watch. I had the feeling that my improvement was considered minor and temporary.

Supporting that view were the blood tests—especially my hematocrit levels—and the symptom of blood in my stools, which my doctors saw as proof that the disease was still raging inside me. They suspected that it might be small quantities of blood being released from my digestive tract as the tumor progressed through my small intestine. My medical record reveals that my physicians found this symptom "worrisome" and "troubling." But, since there was nothing that could be done for me at that point, they decided to leave the problem alone until other symptoms, probably far more severe and revealing, manifested themselves.

I didn't know how to make sense of the blood in the stool. Perhaps it was still a vestige of the cancer. Perhaps it was also a discharge of sorts. I realized that this was rationalizing something that could have been a very severe problem. But the truth was that I was so far gone—at least as far as medicine was concerned—and so little could be done for me, I decided that it was appropriate to rationalize this symptom as much as I needed to. What else could I do? I had to have faith.

Occasionally I spoke to Dr. Angermeier, if for no other reason than to talk with a medical person who still had an open mind. As before, Dr. Angermeier encouraged me to stay on the macrobiotic diet. "From what I see, Marlene, you are making remarkable progress," she told me. "You are not experiencing any of the symptoms we might ordinarily see in a patient with your disease. There's no proof that the macrobiotic diet is helping you, of course. We must admit that your improvement may be attributable to unknown causes that are not related to macrobiotics. But there's an old saying, 'If it ain't broke, don't fix it.' Let's stay the course you're on and continue to monitor your progress closely."

Strengthen the Body and Mind and Let Them Do the Rest

During the first week in June, I decided I wanted to start weight training. The thought had been planted in my mind back in March, when just after I came out of surgery, a friend suggested that I do some light weight training to regain some of the muscle mass I had lost. I asked Dr. Cosimi when I could begin such an exercise routine. At least eight weeks, he told me. That would give my surgical wounds sufficient time to heal.

I wanted to do whatever I could to regain some of my strength, and weight training seemed like a good idea. It was now eight weeks after my surgery, and my scar tissue seemed to be healing nicely.

I went to the Body Lab, a free-weights studio in Providence, where I met Jan Wilson, the owner and primary trainer. She was thin and fit—she had a black belt in karate, I learned later—but more important to me, she was upbeat and supportive. I told her that I had been battling cancer and when she asked me what I was doing for myself, I answered that I had been practicing macrobiotics.

"That's great," Jan said. "For years I practiced macrobiotics, too. I've sort of gone astray," she said, with a sly smile. "But I still try to eat as well as I can.

"Anyway, let's start you out with some light weights. Why don't we try the five-pound weights and see how they feel."

With that, Jan handed me a small barbell. Once it was in my hand, it sank immediately toward the floor, taking my arm with it.

"Wow," said Jan. "Okay. We need something lighter. What about this hollow bar. This is two pounds. How does that feel?"

Jan handed me the hollow barbell. I grasped it with two hands and managed to hold it up. I let it drop slowly and then pulled it up toward my chest.

"I think I can manage this one okay," I said.

"Good," Jan said, smiling supportively. "We'll start out with the bar. We can do all we need to do with just the bar for now."

I met Jan twice a week. Depending on how I felt, we would do anywhere from fifteen to thirty minutes of exercise with the bar.

My attitude was to make myself as strong as I possibly could, using every method I could think of. I completely adopted the macrobiotic view: The body could heal itself. Just give it what it needs to overcome the illness.

Once a week I got a massage from a woman who specialized in Swedish massage and shiatsu, the Japanese form of acupressure. She worked on me very gently for about a half hour to forty-five minutes. I did a half-hour session of yoga twice a month with an instructor and tried to do a short yoga session at home every day. As with the massage, the yoga was very gentle, in part because I tired quickly. But more important, I was told by both my massage practitioner and yoga instructor that if I didn't go slowly and gently, I might actually weaken the healing forces within me. Massage and yoga could break down fat cells, which hold toxins within them, my instructors told me. Once those toxins were released into the bloodstream, they could promote the cancer. On the other hand, gentle massage and yoga would strengthen my organs, especially the blood-cleansing organs, and promote the speedier elimination of disease. I had to be patient. The goal was to promote healing, not force it.

That was among the fundamental lessons of my healing. I had to learn to listen and to be open to opportunities that came to me in their own time. I couldn't just pop a pill or have an operation and instantly be healed. No, my entire understanding of healing was different. Healing was incremental and slow. It was the result, I believed, of grace. For me, grace is the energy that comes to us as a blessing from the divine source. Traditional healers use different terms for grace—in Japan, it is known as *ki;* in China, *Qi,* or chi; in India, *prana,* and in Greece, *pneuma.* No matter what they call it, though, grace is seen as central to the healing process.

Each culture has its own word, and theory that attempts to explain grace, or the essence of life, but all see it as an energy, or force, that flows within each of us and animates our lives. Once that life force leaves the body at time of death, the body ceases to exist and instantly begins to decay. The body no longer possesses the underlying energy that makes it possible for physical organs, cells, and tissues to function. The life force is the basis for our physical existence.

Twice a month, the Providence East West Center had one or another longtime macrobiotic teacher lecture on the subject of healing. The two teachers who came most often were Marc Van Cauwenberg and Ed Esko, a very experienced teacher and protégé of Michio Kushi, the leading macrobiotic teacher in the world. Both Marc and Ed spoke at length about *Qi* as the basis for all healing, and even for all life.

Qi, the two made clear, was a living energy that flowed throughout the universe. Energy is the basis for both health and life. Just as energy is infinitely abundant, it is also infinitely available to all of us. Our capacity to receive and imbibe *Qi* depends on the maturity of our consciousness, or spirit, which in turn determines our awareness of life, our degree of openness and clarity, and our ability to love.

Qi is the energy generated by the earth's rotation, which sends energy generated upward, and by the cosmic bodies, such as the sun, moon, planets, and stars, which send the energy down to the earth in cosmic rays. Every living and inanimate thing on earth is being showered by such energy.

In the Chinese and Japanese healing tradition, energy flows in fourteen pathways, or channels, that traverse the human body and bring *Qi* to every organ, tissue, and cell. The human body uses this energy as the basis for its survival. Along these pathways are thousands of acupuncture points, which act as tiny batteries, boosting *Qi* flow as it moves along these pathways.

In Chinese acupuncture, these fourteen pathways are known as meridians. Each meridian provides *Qi* to specific parts of the body, as well as specific organs, such as the liver or gallbladder or heart. Ten of these meridians bear an organ's name: the heart meridian, the small intestine meridian, the spleen meridian, the stomach meridian, the lung meridian, the large intestine meridian, the kidney meridian, the bladder meridian, the liver meridian, and the gallbladder meridian. The remaining four send energy to groups of organs and coordinate organ functions. They are called the triple heater meridian, the governing vessel, conception vessel, and circulation meridian.

Ideal health is brought about by the unimpeded, or optimal, flow of *Qi* throughout the body and specifically to the organs and tissues served by each of these fourteen meridians. As the energy is restricted, or reduced, organs are deprived of what they need most: energy, or life force.

Our behavior and our thinking determine how effectively and abundantly *Qi* flows within us. Among the most important factors that regulate the amount of *Qi* is how we eat and our degree of physical activity. Just as important, perhaps even more so, are how we breathe, what we think, and what we feel.

Those behaviors that most closely aligned us with *Qi*, or grace, formed the basis for spiritual traditions or religion. Originally, religious traditions and laws—the law of Moses, for example or the practices of Buddhism—were intended to describe a way of life that brought us more into harmony with divine laws. Those who lived in harmony with God's laws were imbued with the life force, which not only infused the body, mind, and spirit, but also gave direction and understanding of life itself. All traditional cultures knew this and even revealed it in their art. Both Jesus and the Buddha are depicted as having a golden glow surrounding them. Jesus has a halo and even speaks of having power flowing through him that is capable of going out to others for the purpose of healing.

The recognition of the life force, its healing power, and its intimate connection with divinity, is present in both Eastern and Western philosophy. Among the ways the life force could be strengthened, according to both Eastern and Western traditions, was through a healing diet. Massage, the laying on of hands, prayer, and meditation were powerful tools, as well, for bringing one into closer alignment with the divine and thereby strengthening the life force. As the macrobiotic practitioners had repeatedly told me, it wasn't just a diet I was following, but a spiritual way of life.

Now I depended on the life force to make me well. And I could draw it to me in greater quantities only by opening up to spiritual life. That meant that my health depended on more than mere medicine, but some type of personal transformation.

The Healing in the Feeling

During this period I became a voracious reader, especially of spiritual and inspirational books. Among the books I read were the Bible, *Love, Medicine, and Miracles* by Bernie Siegel, M.D., *Tough Times Never Last, But Tough People Do* by Robert Schuller, *Anatomy of An Illness* by Norman Cousins, and *Getting Well Again* by Carl Simonton, M.D. All of these books increased my awareness of spirit in daily life by increasing my belief in a positive universe. Without realizing it, I had become increasingly negative as I grew older. I believed that people tended to act selfishly, and that life, more often than not, was tragic. I also had completely given up the belief that divinity would intervene in my life or that something truly positive could happen to me. In fact, I believed just the opposite: anything I would derive from life had to be gotten through struggle.

One of the things that jumped out at me the more I read spiritual literature was how each of us must become open, receptive, and willing to listen to the inner voice and be guided in life. Divine inspiration and grace, these books seemed to be saying, come to those who are open to larger possibilities—not so much through initiating one's will, but by taking up opportunities that mysteriously presented themselves. This awakened me once again to the presence of the feminine.

Of course, I did things in exactly the opposite way: I didn't believe in waiting for an opportunity. If an opportunity was to manifest in my life, it would have to be created by me. My life was shaped, I believed, by my own will. Since everything in my life rested on my efforts, it could just as easily fall if I were not completely engaged in whatever I was doing. I had to give myself totally to the project, because everything depended on me. This, of course, resulted in tremendous tension in my body. Both my massage therapist and my yoga instructor commented on how much tension I held within my body. "Marlene, you can't feel very much, nor can you be in touch with your body, if you're in tension all the time."

My massage therapist explained that by spending so much time on the go and in stress, I created tremendous tension in my body, which resulted in a variety of symptoms, among them poor circulation of blood and lymph; blockage of Qi flow to organs and tissues; distress and pain. The more distress you have in your body, she said, the more your mind attempts to disconnect from your body as a way of escaping distress. "In a way, you're rejecting those parts of your body that are in distress. And that leads to illness." This is especially true of those places where you chronically place your tension, she said. For me, it was clearly in my solar plexus, my lower back, and in my lower organs.

"One of the purposes of massage," she said, "is to help you reconnect in a positive way with parts of your body that you've been out of touch with, sometimes for years. When I put my hand on, say, the small of your back or your solar plexus, your mind automatically goes there. If I touch you in a healing and compassionate way, you'll be able to better connect with that part of your body in the same way. I'll be connecting your compassion with the parts of your body that need healing. You'll be able to experience your body in a new and supportive way."

I had been so hard on my body for so many years that it was no wonder it broke down.

The fact that I had taken a leave of absence from my job allowed me the time and energy to mother myself, as it were. For the first time in my life, I was listening to my body and my own inner voice with attentiveness and a certain love. I cared for it with proper foods, with ample rest, with exercise, and with various forms of therapeutic touch. When I pushed too hard, I rested—without guilt or self-criticism, but with a kind of acceptance and approval that one associates with maternal love.

Ironically, this approach actually empowered me. I say "ironically" because one usually associates power with the masculine, but it was the receptive and the feminine qualities that provided me with the means to regain control of my life. Time slowed down. After years of being buffeted by life, I was now attuning myself to the gentle nurturing forces of life. I was developing faith.

I realized that one of the major characteristics I shared with my mother was that we were both constantly struggling for our survival, and that our way to survive was by constantly staying busy.

Faith would have given me some peace. If I had had faith, I

could have surrendered into the hands of the universe, of God, because I would have believed that God would handle whatever troubles I faced.

But my life was constructed in entirely the opposite way: I lived in constant fear of what *might* happen. I was afraid that the sky was about to fall, or the earth beneath my feet about to give way. Beneath all my churchgoing and respect for the traditions of my religion, beneath the veneer of faith, there was a terrible fear that controlled and drove my life. It was the source of my physical, emotional, and mental tension. It was the source of pain and even of my disease.

The origin of that fear, no doubt, was in my childhood. My father's death, if it was not the actual source, was certainly the moment that that fear took complete control of my life. That's when my mind took over my life completely and buried my heart. That's when I developed the belief that my survival depended on my endless strategies for avoiding danger and difficulties.

If I was to get well, I realized I had to go beyond my current view of the world. I had to develop real faith. Faith that God would protect and provide for me and those I loved. He had the only plan that mattered—that was the only thing that could give me some sense of safety. My life, the outcome of my disease, rested exclusively in His hands.

In confronting my lack of faith, I realized that I had reached the borderline between my family conditioning and a new life. This life of fear was my family pattern, handed down through God knows how many generations. That fear, like a sickness, gripped our family, and then got hold of me. My fate was sealed unless I surrendered, unless I learned to listen and follow. My only hope rested with the thing I feared the most: loss of control.

I prayed constantly now—not only for healing, but for faith. I realized that I wanted to change my life, to return to a saner existence. In the midst of one prayerful session, an idea illuminated my mind. I experienced a tremendous need for purpose. I wanted to have some reason to go on living beyond simply existing for whatever number of years I could possibly extend my life. I needed to know in my heart that my survival mattered to someone else. I wanted my life to affect someone else positively and directly.

No sooner had that need arisen than another revelation flashed within my mind. And in that instant I made a silent promise to myself, and to God. If I were allowed to live, I would try to have another child. Being a mother was the one thing I had done in my life that required unconditional love and unselfish giving. Being a mother put me in a circle of nurturance that I always loved, but seemed to be running away from for years. Yet that love was the surest path I could see to God.

If I survived, I would return life for life. I dedicated myself to the path of the mother. I promised myself that I would mother myself and would give that mothering to a child, if I survived.

A few days later, I had a dream in which I held a baby boy whose name was Joseph Matthew. I awoke from that dream in a state of such exhilaration that I could hardly contain my excitement. The dream was a kind of confirmation. It was as if a postcard had been sent back to me from high above, telling me that my prayer—and my promise—had been heard.

I kept both the promise and the dream a secret, even from Keven. But I held it in my heart, as I did the spirit who might be waiting to join me, a spirit whose name was Joseph Matthew.

CHAPTER 8

Real Progress, With a Little Help from My Friends

Throughout the summer I was well ensconced in my daily health routine. My health habits had become a kind of cocoon from which I hoped to transform myself from a sickly caterpillar to a beautiful, healthy, and vibrant butterfly. Twice a week I worked with Sun to prepare macrobiotic meals. Each day I either reheated Sun's food, or prepared fresh macrobiotic dishes, or combined my own cooking with Sun's. I also prepared standard American fare for my children, sneaking fresh vegetables or some brown rice into their meals whenever I could do it covertly. I still had cravings, especially for sugar, but I resisted them as much as I could. Marc had allowed me a few raisins whenever the cravings became overwhelming. I would put a small mound of raisins in my hand and eat them one at a time, chewing each raisin until I got every ounce of sweetness from it that I could. When the mound of raisins was gone, I was usually satisfied.

Twice a week I lifted weights with Jan and once a week got a massage. Meanwhile, I read a continuous stream of books that uplifted my spirits or made life sensible to me. Several of those books inspired me to begin using positive imaging routines, which I included with my daily prayer sessions.

One of the visualization techniques was to see a beacon of light enter the top of my head and gradually fill up my entire body and soul with warm, healing light. The light radiated from God's hands and entered my being at the crown of my head. It slowly illuminated my head, neck, and shoulders, swirling gently and powerfully as it filled my head, swirling again in my neck, and once more as it filled both my shoulders. It flowed down my arms like liquid gold and streamed into my fingers until it burst from them as smaller beacons of light. From my neck and shoulders, it permeated every cell in my chest and torso. I saw the light pour down through my esophagus, down into my stomach, and then snake through my small intestine. I saw it transform my organs into vibrant, healthy tissue. From there, it went down into my large intestine, reproductive organs, and down my legs, healing every cell as it moved. It swirled at my knees and then streamed through my calves. It swirled again at my ankles and then flowed through my feet, illuminating every toe. From the bottoms of my feet, the light headed downward into the earth, pouring healing energy deep into the core of the planet. As it made its way down into the earth, the light suddenly became a hollow beacon, allowing healing energy to flow back up through me from the earth itself. Earth's force streamed through me like a rushing river, cleansing any vestige of darkness left behind by the downstreaming light.

Whenever I did this technique with real concentration, I was left feeling blessed, relaxed, and restored. For several minutes, sometimes even for more than an hour, I felt as if I were in a state of grace. I tried to do this exercise every morning with my early prayers and sometimes in the evening, as well.

One day, at the end of July, a very strange sensation came over me as I drove to the Body Lab to do my regular workout.

The feeling was so odd that I decided to pull over to the side of the road and rest for a minute. Suddenly I felt utterly relaxed and at peace. A feeling of complete tranquillity and warmth came over me. Out of nowhere came the strong thought—or was it the knowledge?—that I was going to survive. It was as if something almost chemical seeped into my brain and provided some knowledge that had not been there before.

Later, I interpreted this to be the Holy Spirit, who enveloped me and gave me this knowledge, but in that moment there were no lights, no words. There was only the overwhelming sense of harmony and the powerful knowledge that somehow I was going to make it. From that day forward, I had a deep confidence that all that I was doing was working.

In light of my earlier condition, when I was on the verge of death, my growing strength and vitality were nothing short of a miracle. I felt stronger than I had since well before my symptoms had become acute, way back in early 1985. I had more vitality than ever. I slept better and woke up refreshed. Most remarkable, at least to me, I had begun to regain some weight. I was now inching closer to 100 pounds and feeling stronger in my body. My skin was soft and clear. I no longer had dark circles nor big bags of puffy flesh under my eyes. I looked in the mirror and saw a stronger person. If the life force was the basis for existence, health, and healing, then I had more life force in me than I had had in years. I could see it in my eyes and feel it in my body. Energy flowed in me now; I, for one, could not deny it.

I was certain that my improvement would be of great interest to my doctors. Wasn't it obvious that something good was happening to me?

Much to my amazement, most of the physicians I consulted continued to dismiss macrobiotics—and more important, my progress—with a perfunctory wave of the hand. The blood in the stool continued to be troubling to them—"worrisome," according to their reports.

What I came to realize was, in the end, I had to respect my own judgment of my health. I was learning more and more about my body. Indeed, this was one of the primary lessons of my cancer. My progress was based less on what my physicians had done for me than on what I had done for myself. I had to respect and honor that truth. I was the one who was responsible for my health now. I had been the one who had decided to take up macrobiotics, along with half a dozen other health-promoting methods. I had to be the final judge as to whether or not these methods were working. More than at any other time in my life, I was assuming responsibility—not only for my health and happiness, but for my very life.

Of course, I had lots of help.

I would have been utterly alone were it not for a handful of people who embraced me and kept me going forward, especially at my darker moments when fear arose inside me and held me frantic in its grip. Among those who were most helpful to me were Evelyn Rachko, my neighbor who worked in our local hospital's ER. Evelyn continued to come to my house regularly and helped me whenever or wherever she could. Sometimes she even helped me prepare my meals. Macrobiotics was as foreign to Evelyn as the dark side of the moon, but she never ceased to be interested in, and supportive of, my diet. She even tried some of the foods, with varying degrees of success. I remember her telling me that she became interested in daikon radish after I told her that macrobiotic healers believed that daikon could help dissolve masses within the body and that it could be used as an effective diuretic. One day Evie, as I called her, had some friends over for lunch and decided to cover her salad-and-cottage cheese with daikon shavings.

"Marlene, I could barely carry on a conversation because I had to run to the bathroom a half-dozen times that afternoon," she told me, laughing. "All my lady friends were poking fun at me about getting old and having to pee constantly.

'No, no,' I told them. 'It's from the daikon, the white radish I put on my salad.'

" 'Oh, sure,' they said to me.

"But you know what, Marlene, it really works.' " With that, we both burst out laughing.

Of all the people who helped me, Dr. Marc Van Cauwenberg and Eileen Shea were the most important. Were it not for these two people, I would have been cut off from expert advice, experience, and macrobiotic care. They offered a counterweight to the medical world and its stubborn, and even pernicious, skepticism. When my doctors looked at me, they saw a walking anomaly, a contradiction to their experience with cancer, one that no doubt would soon correct itself. Eventually, I would take a turn for the worse and begin my short slide toward death, or so they thought. But with Marc and Eileen, I had two people who not only believed in the power of macrobiotics to heal my disease, but also believed in me and my ability to reverse my condition. Whenever questions arose about some recent symptom or apparent discharge, I called Eileen Shea first. She offered wise counsel, many years of experience, inspiration, and hope. Any question that Eileen couldn't answer, I posed to Marc, who was, for me, the ideal healer. He was a medical doctor, and therefore understood all the medical concerns that came with my disease, and an expert in macrobiotics and traditional Chinese medicine. He embodied the best of both worlds. I considered his presence in my life a miracle all its own.

And finally, there was Keven, my husband. One of the great gifts Keven gave me was his faith in the macrobiotic philosophy and approach to health. After we were on the diet for a while, Keven never looked back. He ate with me every night and went every Friday to our community dinners. In fact, he was so happy to eat the food that it soon became apparent to me that Keven was somehow suited for this diet. If left on a deserted island with nothing to eat but macrobiotic staples, Keven would have been perfectly content. He would never have missed hamburgers and French fries and beer. He loved the food and philosophy and saw the universality of its spiritual truths.

Yet, Keven's approach to macrobiotics was a puzzling set of contradictions. Despite his appreciation for the entire approach, he was also just as content to eat junk food. And much to my dismay, this apparent contradiction was completely lost on him. When he sat down to a macrobiotic meal, he ate the food with true enjoyment and enthusiasm, just as he did when he sat down in front of a hamburger or hot dog. He could exist quite happily with both types of foods as part of his world. In the end I saw his universal palate as a reflection of his innate strength—a kind of appreciation for everything—and, at the same time, an unwillingness to apply the macrobiotic principles to his health and life. Perhaps because he was never really sick, macrobiotics never really got under his skin. While he loved the philosophy of yin and yang, or what George Ohsawa had called "the unique principle," and even felt a kind of kinship with it, Keven never fully embraced the macrobiotic philosophy as his own. The reason, I came to believe, was that the niche within his spirit where he might have placed macrobiotics was already taken up by his Roman Catholicism. Keven's spiritual perspective was defined by his Catholic heritage. And even as he came to truly appreciate macrobiotics, it never became his compass, either philosophically or as a guide to his eating habits. For him, macrobiotics was ultimately a foreign philosophical discipline, beautiful to be sure, but not one that he ever connected to personally.

I took a very different approach. I was just as wedded to my religious traditions, but unlike Keven, I embraced and assimilated macrobiotics into my spiritual life. I imagined that all spiritual traditions taught dietary and health principles—certainly the evidence was all there in the Bible to support such an idea. If anything, macrobiotics enriched my practice of Catholicism because it gave me a fuller appreciation of how I could use food to strengthen my health and grow closer to God.

However, more important than any kind of intellectual or philosophical understanding was my innate practicality: God had sent macrobiotics into my life, and I would have been a completely ungrateful and stupid human being were I to refuse this gift.

Another of my helpers, of course, was Sun Kim, who made it possible for me to eat macrobiotically. Sun and I had developed a warm friendship. But one day late that summer, Sun told me that she and her family were moving away from the area and that she would have to stop cooking for me. By that time I already knew the basics—she had brought me that far—but I was very sorry and even a little afraid to see her go. I still didn't trust myself to prepare my own meals, especially food that I depended on to help me get well. I needed help. And then one night, a beautiful, young woman, thirty-five years old, approached me and asked if she could cook for me. Her name was Christine Scholes, who started cooking for me in August of 1986.

Christine had long, curly brown hair, big brown eyes, and an oval face with high cheekbones. She smiled and laughed easily and often. Christine radiated a kind of relaxed grace and a free-spirited attitude. For many years she owned a natural-foods restaurant in Providence and now taught cooking classes in the Greater Providence area. She had come to macrobiotics only eight years before we met. The reason: She was battling brain cancer. Apparently, she had set some kind of record for the longest-lived patient with her type of disease. Her mother had died of the same kind of brain cancer, and Christine had committed herself to overcoming her disease.

Despite her illness, or perhaps in some way because of it, Christine was absolutely dedicated to helping people with macrobiotics. She was regularly bringing food to those who needed it and had several gravely ill clients for whom she cooked. After learning of all she was doing for people, Keven commented to people privately that he thought she was the closest thing in the community to a saint. To my infinite good fortune, I was the latest person on whom she bestowed her love and blessing.

Twice a week she would come to my house and prepare my meals for the week ahead. Unlike Sun, with whom I fumbled through the food preparation, Christine was a professional chef, an expert. She glided through the kitchen, bringing the power of her personality to every meal she made. The staple foods—the grains, vegetables, beans, and soups—that had been so ordinary and bland were now intensified in flavor, color, and presentation. Christine always presented something exotic in addition to her brown rice, collard greens, and carrots. She made *seitan*—wheat gluten—that had a rich, savory flavor and a consistency that chefs strive for when preparing the most tender steak. She made shish kebobs with sautéed vegetables, cut thick, along with tofu and *seitan*, covered with her own special sauce. She made quiches from grains, vegetables, and a little flour; tender and heavenly fish; sauces that turned otherwise bland foods into entrees that you couldn't help going back to for more. This was restaurant flavor with medicinal quality. Even the seaweed was delicious.

Needless to say, I provided only minimal assistance in the kitchen. On the contrary, I watched Christine with a certain awe. It amazed me that this thin, gentle person could command so much space, and with such authority. And the food! She had a gift for cooking and for helping people. But even more, she had a way of giving to people without ever burdening others with the knowledge that she was ill herself. Christine never let on—at least not in her manner—that she was battling a life-threatening cancer. On the contrary, she seemed loath to appear weak or dependent. Instead of being needy, she helped those who needed others. Even her self-lessness was unobtrusive.

Occasionally the cancer would trigger a seizure. The attacks would force her to rest, usually for a day or two, and sometimes longer. During these periods she would take to her bed. Eileen Shea or some other member of the community might bring her food. Yet in no time she would be out of bed and back at her cooking jobs.

In addition to cooking, Christine practiced yoga regularly and was the one who introduced me to the practice. I was so stiff when I started! My body was all tied in knots. Was I even *in* my body most of the time? I wondered. I asked that question because I had begun to realize that most of the time I lived in my head, ruminating about the future or the past. Rarely did I actually focus on the present and what I was doing at this particular moment. Yoga changed that, at least for the thirty minutes I did it each day. All I could concentrate on were the postures and the pain I experienced from stretching muscles that hadn't been stretched in decades. How wonderful it was, though, to be brought back to the absolute *now* and the simplicity of an ordinary movement. I sat on the floor and reached for my knee or toe. I lay on my back and reached upward with my pelvis. With deliberate concentration, I maintained my balance as I stood on one foot and reached up with both hands clasped. Through yoga I became aware of what it meant to merely *be*.

Sometimes, while the instructor was leading us, I would look over at Christine and watch her as she moved gracefully and gently into a posture. Like me, Christine was living under the cloud of a death sentence. Watching her perform yoga or cook, I became aware of how committed she was to living in the now and enjoying as much of her life as she could. Only by living in the present can we truly be free of fear, I realized. Christine was teaching me that. She performed her yoga exercises with perfect concentration on the present moment. She was teaching me not to watch anyone else, not to focus on anything but my own inner life. Turn inward, she seemed to be saying, and spend whatever amount of time you have left learning about who you are. I would resume my exercises, focused with renewed energy. Yoga was meditation in action, just as life should be.

New Signs of Health

It was sometime in early September, about a month after Christine started cooking for me, when I realized I was no longer producing cysts and tumors on my body. In fact, it seemed to me that many of the tumors and cysts had actually receded and disappeared. What was happening to me? Were the underlying conditions that supported my cancer receding, as well? Surely, that must be the case. Maybe I don't have cancer anymore, I thought. It was as if the thought had suddenly taken hold of me. Hope and desire rose within me like a geyser. Could it be true? It's possible, I thought. Oh, God, let it be so. But with hope came its inevitable brother, fear, which engulfed me now. What if it's not true, I said to myself. What if I still do have cancer! I now realized that in a very odd way I had come to expect my health to return. The diet and spirituality had been working so powerfully that some unspoken and largely unconscious part of me expected to get well. No doubt, that part of me had tossed up the thought that I had already defeated the cancer. That hopeful, intuitive, and inspirational side stood in the face of my rational mind, which is rife with fear. Now I feared that my sudden inspiration might be nothing more than false hope, and that the cancer might be spreading at this very moment.

All of the calm and contentment, which soothed me just seconds before, were gone now. In their places were internal conflict and tumult. I wanted so badly to believe that it wasn't just my own wishful thinking that had caused this thought to emerge. I wanted to believe that some inner wisdom was speaking to me from deep within. I was feeling better physically and emotionally—that was a fact, I told myself. And yes, I had made a miraculous turnaround in only four months. But aside from my physical symptoms and the small evidence of my blood tests—the results of which had made little impression on my doctors—there was no objective proof that I was, in fact, healthier. Even the fact that I was no longer producing tumors on the surface of my skin meant nothing to my doctors. They believed that the disease had moved inside me now and was ravaging my intestines. Indeed, my doctors kept focusing on the small amount of blood that had been found in my stool sample as proof of such speculation.

Perhaps they were right, I thought. They had so much more knowledge and experience than I did. What could I possibly know? What could any of these macrobiotic people know? Granted, Marc was a medical doctor, but he might also be a kook.

But at the end of the month, my blood tests made a radical improvement, as well. In fact, all of them were now normal.

Ever since my discharge from Massachusetts General Hospital in March, I had been having monthly blood tests to monitor my condition. Those tests were expected to reveal progressive disease. Instead, my liver tests, particularly SGOT and alkaline phosphatase, were both normal. Other liver tests, such as bilirubin, which was abnormally high before and after my surgery, were also normal now. More important, both my hemoglobin and my hematocrit levels were normal for the first time since way before my surgery. I was no longer anemic and had a normal red-blood-cell count.

When those tests came back normal, I cried with joy. I was definitely feeling stronger and had more energy than I had had in many months. Now my blood tests revealed a distinct improvement in my condition. I wasn't just imagining progress—there was proof! I couldn't believe it. I had only been practicing macrobiotics since the first week in May and now, just five months later, I was showing definite and definable signs of improvement.

In early October my dermatologist noted that my skin had noticeably improved. In an October 8, 1986, letter to my internist, he stated, "To my gross examination, there was no clinical evidence of disease. There were no new suspicious pigmented lesions, no subcutaneous masses, no adenopathy, and no organomegaly that I could detect."

My doctors were always quick to follow up such signs of improvement with the expectation of disease. As my dermatologist wrote in his letter: "This, of course, does not preclude that she has continued growth of the internal lymph glands and additional metastases to her bowel, which is producing the occult positive blood that you are now detecting."

While my doctors refused to fully acknowledge my improvement, I was jumping for joy. There was one test left to do to determine if in fact there was cancer left inside me. That was to undergo a magnetic resonance imaging test, or MRI. I told my doctor to schedule such a test for late in October. By then, I believed, I could show that I was well.

CHAPTER 9

The Light at the End of the Tunnel

Once I decided to have the MRI, I couldn't wait to know. I had to have more objective evidence that I was indeed making progress.

I telephoned Marc Van Cauwenberg and asked him what he thought of the test.

"The human body runs by electromagnetic energy," he said. "The body is an electrical system." He went on to explain that health is the result of a natural harmony within that electrical system, a harmony that allows electromagnetic energy, or *Qi*, as he put it, to flow to every cell and organ in one's body.

Marc explained that every function within the body, even the tiniest cellular activity, relies on a balanced flow of electromagnetic energy. "We are living in an infinite electrical field," Marc said. "At the same time we're trying to harmonize with that field."

An MRI, Marc said, could be destructive to health because it could interfere with the body's electrical balance and its attempts to take in and harmonize with the large energy flowing to us from heaven and earth. "I cannot make the decision for you," Marc said. "I can only express my concerns about the test. You have to make the decision."

"I have to know, Marc," I said. "Something inside of me tells me that I'm well, but every time I allow myself to believe I'm getting better, I start to have doubts and fears. I need some kind of objective measure that shows I'm improving."

"Then do what you think is best," he said. He then gave me an array of dietary recommendations to support my body when I underwent the test, including eating seaweed daily, which would provide an abundance of minerals that would support my electrical system; lots of leafy green vegetables, which were also rich in minerals; and finally, lots of brown rice to strengthen and balance my nervous system, which no doubt would be affected by the MRI.

"Let's see each other after you have the test," he said.

In October my doctor scheduled a magnetic resonance imaging test that we hoped would give us a good idea of my state of health. As his letter indicated, my doctor told me in advance that he expected to find tumors scattered throughout my small intestine. In effect, the test would reestablish what Dr. Cosimi, my surgeon at Massachusetts General Hospital, had found when he opened my small intestine and found cancerous tumors spread throughout the organ.

Keven and I arrived early for our 9 A.M. appointment at Miriam Hospital in Providence, where we met the doctor and a nurse who would administer the test. I was then led to an inner room, in the middle of which sat the MRI machine.

The magnetic resonance imaging machine is essentially a long cylinder that is open at both ends. Protruding at one end is a trough, or bed, on which the patient lies and is then moved into the cylinder. In the same room where the machine is located, a television monitoring device presents the images the machine detects. This allowed Keven and my doctor to view the results of my test as it was taking place.

The nurse assisted me in getting onto the troughlike bed. Once I was in position, she pushed a button on the side of the MRI machine and a conveyorlike system moved my body into the cylinder. The cylinder seemed little more than three feet wide; it was tighter all around me than I had expected. The interior of the cylinder was shiny metal. At my feet I could see the opening by which I entered.

I immediately became claustrophobic and afraid. Hoping to forestall panic, I started to pray to the Holy Mother. Suddenly the machine came alive and started to whir. My heart, which had been beating like a terrified rabbit, now jumped in my chest. I could feel it pounding in my rib cage and hear it in the vessels of my ears. I prayed with a terrible intensity and fought the fear that seized me.

The machine itself works by using a powerful electromagnetic field in combination with radio signals to detect changes in hydrogen atoms, which are the most numerous kind of atoms in the body. A pooling of hydrogen atoms, for example, may indicate the presence of disease.

The MRI machine has the power to "see" through bone, but has the sensitivity to delineate numerous types of changes in tissue. It can detect, for example, something as seemingly subtle as edema, or fluid retention, and as thick as scar tissue, such as that which forms in the heart muscle after a heart attack. It can also reveal the presence of tumors.

The information flowing from the MRI is sent to a video monitor, which translates that information into television images. It is also transferred to film, which doctors and technicians can read later on.

The test itself takes as much as ninety minutes, which meant that I was forced to lie there, terrified, for what seemed like a lifetime. What would this machine come to symbolize for me? Would it confirm the presence of cancer throughout my small and large intestine, as my doctors suspected. In that case, the machine would be a metallic grave. Or would it reveal what I hoped, what my spirit cried out for, that I was free of cancer, in which case it would be a chrysalis, my cocoon, from which I would emerge reborn.

Right now, however, this machine communicated nothing more to me than cold objectivity. It held me in its womb without a trace of love or caring. It was merely curious about me, nothing more. I was to be punctured and dissected by its invisible waves, held indifferently within the cold embrace of its magnetic field. I was nothing—just a body that fed the beast information, which it would relay back to my doctor.

Ever since I had put on this hospital gown, I had been cold. Now I was shivering. The nurse had asked me not to move because it blurred the images that were transferred to the video screen. I tried to relax and hold still.

Suddenly the whirring sound changed to clicks and then back to whirring. Oh, Mother Mary, what did this thing detect? What was it telling my doctor? Protect me.

Finally the whirring stopped and the machine became lifeless. Now the conveyor belt sounded and my body was slowly drawn from the cylinder. As I moved back into the world of the living, I looked at my doctor, who was businesslike and impassive, and then at Keven, who smiled happily at me. At that moment I knew. My heart, which had begun to slow down after the machine stopped, was suddenly jumping again—this time, with hopeful and excited anticipation.

"Why don't you get dressed, Marlene, and we'll talk," my doctor said.

I hurried behind the curtain and quickly threw on my clothes. I was still putting myself back together when I emerged. "We'll go into my office," my doctor said.

When we got there, he sat down behind his desk, while Keven and I sat on the two chairs that stood before it.

"Marlene, your MRI shows no signs of cancer," my doctor announced. "This is not conclusive proof of anything, of course, but it certainly is a good sign. As I have told you, there are also no visible signs of cancer on your body that I can detect. Your blood tests are all normal. There was the single test revealing some blood in the stool, which I find worrisome, but don't really know what to make of at this point. Apart from that test, you seem in good health. This doesn't mean that the cancer will not grow back," he said. "But for the moment, I cannot find any cancer in your body."

I clasped Keven's hand and said, "Thank you, Doctor." I closed my eyes momentarily and thanked God. I was jubilant inside. I was not prepared to share too much with my doctor, however, for fear that he might feel compelled to say things that would, in essence, throw a bucket of cold water on my enthusiasm.

He asked me if I had any questions. I couldn't think straight. "Wouldn't you say that this was fairly out of the ordinary?" I blurted out.

He knew where this was headed. In the past he always resisted any conversation involving macrobiotics. "Well, we don't know yet, because I just don't know how to interpret your test results," he answered. "We cannot draw any firm conclusions, one way or the other. As I said, these results do not mean that the cancer will not come back."

I did not want the conversation to go any further. I turned and smiled at Keven and said, "Well, I guess that's it. Let's go."

Back from the dead, I thought later that day. I was exuberant. Nothing in my life had ever given me a greater feeling of joy and enthusiasm for life. I had rejoined the living. But it wasn't just because a test had given me a clean bill of health. The test was mere confirmation. What mattered even more was the way I felt. I had strength, energy, clarity of thought and emotion. I felt good in body and soul.

That afternoon when all my children—except Sean, whom I would telephone later that day—came home from school, I gathered them around me and told them the good news. I had become so practiced at keeping the whole truth from them that even now I had trouble confessing how grave my situation was.

"You know, for a long time I was very sick, sicker than I was even telling you all," I said to them. "But for the past several months, I have been taking good care of myself and eating that crazy diet that you guys like to make so much fun of. And today I had a test and my doctor told me that I am fine. And I'm so happy that I just wanted to tell you all that."

"That's great, Mom," Christopher said. "What kind of test did you have?"

I explained the MRI and told them a little about the experience, especially the claustrophobia.

"Were you scared?" Mary Kathryn asked, concern radiating from her eyes.

"Oh, yes, I was very afraid," I said.

"Does this mean that you don't have to eat that seaweed anymore?" Damian asked.

I laughed. "No, it doesn't, Damian. I'm going to eat that seaweed for the rest of my life. I have even come to like it. And you know what, I'm well now because of that seaweed and all the other foods I've been eating these past five months. Someday, I hope that you'll eat that way, too."

"No way," Damian said. We all laughed. "Some of the foods are all right," he added, "but I like hamburgers."

"I know. But let's not talk about food anymore. Let me just hug you all and tell you how much I love you."

With that, the four of us did a group hug. "Why are you crying?" Mary Kathryn asked me.

"I'm just happy, that's all, honey."

That November, we had a big Thanksgiving dinner, which Christine and I prepared for thirty members of my family, including my mother and my brother Al and his wife. The meal was entirely vegetarian, but it was an enormous feast. Christine outdid herself, making the most incredible macrobiotic party food: great quantities of *seitan,* covered with a wide variety of sauces—some sweet and sour, others savory and rich; her own bread stuffing, mounds of mashed sweet potatoes, six or eight exotic vegetable dishes, including numerous orange and yellow squashes, a big bowl of brown rice, fried noodles with mushrooms and vegetables, and a beautiful squash soup. The meal was an explosion of color that equaled autumn at its peak of pigmented beauty.

We all sat down, looked at one another with deep gratitude, and gave thanks. And even Damian loved the food that day.

What next? I thought as I watched the family dive into this beautiful meal. I couldn't imagine ever being happier.

CHAPTER 10

Birth and Rebirth

The months that followed my MRI and blood tests were something like being on work-release from prison. I was free from the immediate fears and the debilitation of my disease. I had energy and time again, the essence of life. That experience alone was a miracle. Every day was now a gift, like the fresh arrival of spring. I was happy in every cell of my body. For a time, even the chores of my life were a blessing. Going to the store and making meals for my family were a pleasure, in part because I did those things now without the shadow of death oppressing me. During most of the previous year, there was no escaping that shadow. The mere presence of death and the barely hidden expectation that I would soon be gone were suffocating me. Suddenly I had escaped. I was free.

I experienced that freedom in the oddest moments. I'd be doing the dishes, or walking the aisles in my grocery store, and my mind would wander to my darkest fear. Suddenly the specter of illness and death would engulf me, as it had been doing for most of the previous year. Darkness, in the form of a belief in my own imminent death, would overtake me. And then suddenly, as if the sun had magically appeared, I would realize that I was well. All the tests that I could take had confirmed it. I was well; I was healthy. The illness had been defeated. Joy would swell in my chest, and my eyes would fill with tears. I would be cruising the produce and trying to hide the fact that I was wiping my eyes—with a smile on my face. Such moments were awkward and comical.

Day after day, some form of this little experience repeated itself. Day after day, the sun would come up over the darkened landscape of my inner life. This was the daily gift of life that I had been given.

And yet, this period was not without its shadow. I was well, yes, but I took nothing for granted. I had been sick for too long; I had been too close to the abyss to forget. Death was a reality, if not today, then certainly at some future tomorrow. And then there was the mystery of cancer. Even after I had somehow overcome the illness, I never felt fully free of it. My second mind, the part of me that exists right below my normal consciousness, was still in fear. On some level I had believed what my doctors told me—that even though the signs were good, the cancer could come back. I was on cancer's leash. My health and my freedom were tenuous. They could be yanked away from me at any moment. Therefore, I had to be careful with my eating habits and my lifestyle if I was going to secure my new life.

I decided to give myself the entire year of 1987 to recuperate. I was not going to rush back to work, nor was I going to get back into the stress of my former existence. Of course, this was a financial hardship for us, one that we had been enduring for much of the past year. But there really was no other decision to make. To reenter the investment world and all that stress was tantamount to inviting my cancer to return. Once this decision was made, I was at peace with myself. And as the months passed and my overall health continued to improve, my perception of my vulnerability began to pass. I gained increasing confidence in my body and my future.

In the late autumn of 1987 I felt strong enough to take on some social challenge. I wanted to be of service to people, to do something with the life I had been given. At first I didn't have a clue what I could do. I didn't know enough about macrobiotics to be a teacher and I certainly wasn't qualified to serve people in a spiritual capacity. Yet, I wanted to give something to people that could make their lives better. This, in fact, had always been my dream. Over the years I got side-tracked by life's many demands and burdens, particularly by the need to earn a living and maintain a business. The more deeply I got involved in the business world, the more I got sucked into the struggle to survive. And the more I became preoccupied by my own survival, the more concerned I became about myself and my own problems. I didn't want that to happen again. I reflected for weeks on what I might do. I realized that whatever I decided, my new work would have to come out of my own experience of life. The two things I knew were the world of finance and politics. So late that fall I decided to run for Rhode Island general treasurer, and in January 1988 I announced my candidacy.

Almost instantly I was drawn into the tumultuous world of politics, studying the issues, formulating my positions, building a political organization, meeting the right people, and fund-raising.

A month later, I discovered that I was pregnant.

Initially I was shocked and even amazed. I couldn't believe that I was capable of getting pregnant. I was forty-two years old, certainly young enough to have another baby, but I had just been through cancer. How could my body have the strength to conceive and give birth? Suddenly my promise came to mind. I had promised God that if I survived cancer, I would give birth to another child. In an instant I realized that my pregnancy was yet another confirmation that my prayers had been heard. I knew now that there was someone there listening to every prayer I uttered—and every promise made.

That realization was so profound that it momentarily blotted out everything else in my life. I was alone with God. For a very short time, there were no doubts, no feelings of separation. I was utterly exposed and yet held within that unity. I felt overwhelming love. There were no words to describe that experience. I was consumed in a flame of joy.

My doctors did not have the same reaction, however. The first doctor I consulted was my internist, who advised me that the increased hormonal activity associated with pregnancy could bring back my cancer. Studies had shown that women who were in remission from malignant melanoma and who subsequently became pregnant experienced a recurrence of the disease. She told me in no uncertain terms that if the pregnancy went full term, it could kill me.

I then consulted my dermatologist, who had taken over for Dr. Angermeier and was now following my cancer. He reiterated my internist's concerns, as did my oncologist from Mass General. All three urged me to have an abortion. In fact, abortion was my only choice if I expected to go on living.

The night I was given this news, Keven and I sat in our living room and discussed what we should do. Keven had always been opposed to abortion on principle. He had never imagined that his wife would ever have to face the prospect of having one.

"Who could have conceived of these circumstances?" Keven asked. "These doctors are telling us that we either have an abortion or you die?"

"Do you think it's true, Keven?" I asked.

"Well, let's face it, Marlene, their track record hasn't been all that good. I mean, on the basis of what we've seen so far, I wouldn't bet on their accuracy. On the other hand, what if they're right? You've made all this progress by doing what they told you not to do, but wouldn't it be ironic if we went against them one more time and this time they turned out to be right?!"

"I feel that if I agree to an abortion, it's like making a pact with the devil," I said. "I feel as if I would be killing an innocent life in order to live. How could I live with that?"

I sighed. "Keven, I know what I shouldn't do, but I don't feel any clear direction about what I should do," I said. "I know I can't have the abortion, but I feel so unclear about the future. I want to be clear and certain. I want to feel some conviction about what I'm doing. Right now, I don't. All I feel is fear."

We both agreed that I should sit down in private with our parish priest, Father Marcel Pincince. Perhaps with some spiritual counseling, I could start to get to my answer.

Where All Answers Lie

Father Pincince, the parish priest at Blessed Sacrament Church, was about thirty-five years old, and handsome in a kind of elfish way. He always gave me the impression that he was slightly bouncy, because everything he did seemed to radiate an excess of energy. When he walked, he almost seemed to run. When he stopped and looked at you, he somehow still seemed in motion. He was warm, accepting, and humble. He was also joyful and open to everyone. I called him and told him of my problem. He asked me to come to the rectory and see him the following day.

The next day, we met in a little sitting room. It was early February and the afternoon sun was weak and watery. It seemed to come through the lace curtains in a pale haze. I was restless. As I spoke, I found myself struggling to present the facts in a coolly dispassionate way, as if I could think the problem through and arrive at the only logical conclusion—a conclusion I still could not see.

As I explained my dilemma, Father Pincince listened attentively, occasionally asking me a question when I paused to collect my thoughts. When I was finished, I said that I did not want to have an abortion, but I did not want to go back into the hell that I had just come out of.

"My mother died of breast cancer," Father Pincince said. "It was terrible. She suffered so much. She carried on as best she could, and she really fought, but in the end the disease consumed her. No one wants you to go back into that."

"Keven and I are opposed to abortion, Father," I said. "We definitely believe that it's wrong. But I never dreamed that my belief would require me to choose between an abortion and my life. In an odd way I feel I am being forced by religion and my principles to do something that may kill me."

"You do not have to be forced to do anything," Father Pincince said. "And you mustn't be forced, not if this is to turn out right in the end. There is a right path for you, a path that God wants you to travel, Marlene. But only you can find that path," he told me. "If people say that you should do this or that, and you accept such advice, then you are allowing yourself to be forced into doing something. Then you would be allowing others to make your decision for you.

"This may turn out to be a medical decision. If it is, you must be at peace with that. The only way you can find such peace is if you know in your heart that that is what God wants you to do.

"God's path can only be found by searching your own heart deeply. This is a difficult decision, but there is peace when we know what is right for us and we walk that path. No matter how difficult it becomes, we realize that we choose the path that God wanted us to walk. That is all we can hope for in life.

"I know a place where you can go for the weekend and just pray and meditate. It's called the Mercy Lodge, in Cumberland. The Sisters of Mercy provide a spiritual atmosphere of quiet contemplation. They will also listen to you if you would like to talk. I will make the arrangements for you. Go there, pray, meditate, listen to your heart. God's answer will come to you."

Father Pincince smiled. "Meanwhile, I will pray for you."

I arrived at the Mercy Lodge in Cumberland, Rhode Island, on a Friday afternoon in late February. The lodge itself looked like a big bed-and-breakfast. The main house was a large Victorian that had been divided into smaller bedrooms. I was led to my room by one of the nuns and told that if I wanted to talk during the three days I would be with the sisters, I should seek out Sister Kathleen.

I unpacked my bags and sat down to gaze out the window. The house stood in the middle of acres of open ground. There was snow all around, and in the waning afternoon light everything seemed still and hibernating. Life seemed buried beneath the season. As I looked out onto the wintry landscape, it was hard to believe that spring would ever return. I got up from my chair and went downstairs for a silent dinner and then returned to my room to pray and meditate.

At least, that was my intention. Alone in my room, I was soon enveloped by my fears. The more I thought, the more fear I experienced and the more I wanted an immediate answer. I was so confused. I didn't want to die. I didn't want my cancer to come back. I didn't even want to think about it. Should I have the abortion? I kept asking myself. What should I do? Is there another way? What would it be like to have an abortion? How would I feel? I'd be justified, I told myself. This pregnancy might just be a mistake. How do I know that the child is even healthy? Certainly, I am not fully recovered from all I have been through.

I slept fitfully and woke up an emotional wreck. I spent that Saturday alone and in near hysteria. Thoughts whizzed through my head like opposing bullets. Yes, I should go ahead with the pregnancy. No, I should end the pregnancy and live. How would an abortion affect my marriage? How would Keven feel about me? How could I live with myself?

Such thoughts led to a tumult of emotion. I hated Keven for having such strong feelings. I hated myself for allowing the circumstances to get to this point. Why, God? I kept asking. How could I have made such a promise? I felt like a fool. It was all my fault that I was in this situation. I blamed myself and became even more angry.

Finally that anger gave way to sadness and I broke down in tears. I cried for hours; it felt like days. I realized at some point that I still had grieving to do for all the pain I had been through these past few years. And when I finally was drained of all the tears that I had for this day, I realized that no one was at fault for the situation in which I found myself. This was life. Perhaps it was even grace. I was only seeing the dark side of all of this, I realized. Perhaps there was goodness at the center of this. Of course there is, I thought. There is a child within me, wanting to be born.

The following day, Sunday, I attended early mass and for an hour sat in stillness and meditation. I had expended so much emotion and energy the previous day that now I was empty inside. In that emptiness I felt profound peace and grace. For the first time that weekend, I was relatively free of emotion. In that freedom, clarity descended upon me.

What is the meaning of my life? I kept asking myself. Who or what is the source of my life? Is the medical profession the source of my health, a profession that assured me—once again—that I would soon be dead if I did not follow its counsel? Or is it a higher power that is my source, a power I can turn to in this crisis?

The forces of life within us conspire to make us believe that death will never come. But I had come too close to death to harbor any illusions about death's inevitability. Sooner or later, it would be here. And I didn't have to have a baby to ensure death's arrival. How would I go to God if I broke that promise, I thought. Not fulfilling my promise was tantamount to spiritual death for me, because I would be betraying the very Lord who rescued me before, and on whom I would have to depend to rescue me again.

In some deep place within me, I felt supported. I now believed that I would be all right, whatever I did. Of course, in a way, I already knew what I was going to do, but I wanted to talk to Sister Kathleen first to hear what she had to say.

Sister Kathleen wore a modest blouse and skirt—not the clerical habit that I had grown up seeing nuns wear. Her brown hair was mixed with gray and it fell to below her ears. She was slight of build, but she radiated strength and wisdom.

I told her my story and asked her what she thought I should do.

"When you first started talking, I was on the verge of telling you to go ahead and have an abortion, but right after you finished, this wonderful feeling came over me and I felt very deeply that you were going to be fine. I cannot tell you what to do, but I do believe that if you have the baby, nothing bad will happen to you. I really do have a strong feeling that you and your baby will come out of this healthy and well."

With that, she released this very soft, peaceful smile. And I, too, felt that same wonderful feeling and believed, as she did, that everything would be all right.

"I believe you're right, Sister," I said. "I think it's all going to work out. I'm going to have the baby. And do you know what, I already know his name."

We laughed together and then embraced. Later that afternoon I returned home and told Keven of my decision to go ahead with the pregnancy.

"Are you sure, Marlene?"

"Yes, I'm sure," I said.

My doctors, of course, thought I was crazy, but I could only guess that they had been thinking I was crazy for months now, ever since I began the macrobiotic diet. I had no trouble with them, however, because no one was willing to compel me to have an abortion. They simply remained silent and, as before, waited for my cancer to return. It never did.

Once I made my decision, I was absolutely at peace with myself. One night I gathered all my children together and told them that there would be a new addition to the family. I was going to have a baby, I said. For a moment they were stunned, and then gradually they started to smile and ask me questions.

"That's amazing," Christopher said.

"Wow, Mom," said Damian.

Mary Kathryn looked momentarily confused, but finally was able to formulate her question. "How did that happen?"

Everyone laughed. "We'll talk about it later, but for now you should realize that you're going to have a baby brother or sister."

"I'm not going to be the youngest anymore!" Mary Kathryn said.

"And you're okay? I mean, having a baby is fine and you're okay and all?" Sean asked with more than a hint of concern in his voice.

"I'm fine, Sean. Thank you. And it will be fine," I said. With that, we all hugged and kissed each other.

Of course, there was a steady stream of questions over the months ahead, especially from Damian and Mary Kathryn, who seemed to marvel the most at the steady swelling of my stomach.

Meanwhile, I went back to my campaign for state treasurer, traversing little Rhode Island as if it was my own backyard. The primary elections were held on September 14, 1988, and I pushed hard to win. But I didn't. Ten days later, Keven and I rushed to the hospital where I gave birth to a healthy baby boy, whom I named Joseph Matthew.

"You are my miracle child," I told Joseph as I lay in my

hospital bed on the morning I would be discharged. Keven had not yet arrived and no one was in the room but Joseph and me. Joseph lay in my arms, pink and contented. Something about him made me feel that he was acutely aware of my every breath and my every thought. "Look at you," I whispered to him. "You're beautiful and perfect and you've made me so happy." I snuggled him and kissed his head. "You've come so far and you've been so strong. Nothing was going to stop you, was it? Not those silly doctors, that's for sure. You gave your mom strength. You were up there watching over me and telling me that we were going to be fine. You were whispering in my ear, 'Don't listen to them. Listen to your heart. It knows the way.' And I did. I listened to you and my heart and here we are today, ready to go home to your father and your brothers and sister. You taught me so much already, and you just got here. You're so loved. Do you know that? Yes, I think you do." With that, I kissed his head again.

In December, Joseph was baptized by Father Pincince at the Blessed Sacrament Church. More than one hundred people crowded into the church to celebrate a mass for Joseph's baptism. The church was all lit up in its Christmas colors, and Father Pincince gave a beautiful homily, emphasizing what a miracle Joseph was. Clearly, Father Pincince was moved himself by the event. He smiled often and broadly and he radiated an uplifting energy that seemed to raise everyone in the service to new heights of inspiration and joy. Throughout the mass he used the word "miracle" over and over again in connection with Joseph's birth.

"Sometimes we wonder if miracles happen anymore, or if they can happen to us, but here is a miracle, right in front of us," Father Pincince said. "This child is living proof that God hears our prayers and that miracles do happen when we have faith."

Later, after the mass, Father Pincince conducted the baptism with the same joyful, open heart with which he celebrated the mass. He baptized Joseph with prayer and with water, which he poured over Joseph's head. Joseph let out a little cry and I drew him toward me, kissed his cheek, and whispered in his ear, "This long road has led to you."

Part Two

CHAPTER 11

A Healing Diet and Healing Herbs

The story of my encounter with terminal cancer and ultimate recovery embodies the problems every American faces when dealing with a life-threatening illness and the very real limitations of modern medicine. We must find ways to improve our health, fight our disease, and maintain hope. The guidelines that follow can do all three.

The first section describes the vital role that diet plays in regaining our health. With so many dietary experts today explaining why their diet works better than their competitors, we can easily become confused about what we should eat. Our confusion can be quickly eliminated, however, if we realize that the diets of our ancestors—the foods we humans evolved on—were dominated by plants, with smaller amounts of animal foods. To be sure, our ancient ancestors ate animal foods whenever they could, but such occasions were more haphazard, especially in the Paleolithic period, when our hunting tools were extremely primitive. Also, game tended to run in seasons. Consequently, people relied on plant foods—tubers, fruit, and leafy vegetables, primarily—to sustain themselves.

About thirty thousand years ago, we started to eat wild

grains, and when agriculture was established, about ten thousand years ago, we relied upon cultivated grains as the center of our diet.

A diet composed chiefly of whole grains, fresh vegetables, beans, fruit, and low-fat animal products is the one promoted by virtually every knowledgeable scientist and scientific body. I refer to this diet as a macrobiotic diet, but it is essentially the same as the Pritikin diet and the regimen followed today by most traditional and native populations throughout the world. It also is very similar to the dietary recommendations made by the United States surgeon general.

Until the 1980s, the medical establishment resisted any suggestion of a link between modern diet and degenerative disease. Then in 1982 the National Academy of Sciences reported studies linking diet with between sixty and ninety percent of all cancers. Since that time, there has been a great deal of interest in the connection between food and disease, with science consistently recommending a diet made up of whole grains, fresh vegetables, beans, fruit, and low-fat animal products as the way to both prevent disease and boost the body's own healing mechanisms.

It is clear that the seemingly "miraculous" healing power of food has a solid basis in modern Western science. In fact, scientific research of the past decade is providing ample proof that diet can be a powerful tool for healing. It has been shown, for example, that antioxidants, present in most plant foods, boost the immune system and reverse the course of some diseases. Other elements within foods, especially certain cancer inhibitors, such as phytochemicals and flavonoids, not only prevent cancer but actually attack tumors and cancer cells themselves. Research by the National Cancer Institute and other major scientific centers demonstrates the rational scientific support for the macrobiotic approach to cancer and other illnesses.

Let's look at why these foods are different from all other foods, and better for us. Civilization and community began when people learned to gather and then grow one food in great quantities. That food was grain. Grain allowed people to stop being nomads and to create homes, form organized societies, enact laws, and understand the seasons and weather patterns. They learned agriculture and self-sufficiency. Grain became the basis for stability and orderly living. In Asia the grains were rice, wheat, and barley; in the Middle East it was wheat and barley; in Europe it was wheat, oats, and barley; and in the Americas it was corn, wheat, barley, oats, and later rice.

Since agriculture was the basis of every civilization, the foods most in abundance were grains, vegetables, beans, and fruit. Livestock was extremely expensive. Consequently, meat tended to be eaten in smaller quantities, and only during feasts and celebrations was it the center of the meal and served in larger amounts.

Since grain provided for people's survival, it was regarded as sacred—a food delivered by the gods, or God himself. In virtually every culture grain became intertwined with religion; the endless array of rituals and myths that involve grain are present in virtually every country's heritage. In both Japan and India, for example, it is said that the gods themselves delivered rice and wheat to the people. The Native Americans held similar myths about corn.

We are now going back to the ways of our ancestors. Ironically, it is not religion that is leading us back, but concerns for our health and the overwhelming support of scientific evidence.

Science has shown that at least six of the ten leading causes of death are related to diet. Researchers have demonstrated that diet is associated with, or a causal factor for, heart disease, cancer, adult-onset diabetes, high blood pressure, stroke, overweight, and osteoporosis.

Many argue today that we are living longer than ever before. In fact, the Japanese, the longest-living people on earth, have subsisted on a diet largely of whole grains, vegetables, beans, and low-fat animal products through most of their history. Japanese women live 82.5 years, on average; while the men live to age 76.2. On the longevity ladder, Americans have little to brag about, despite our high-tech medical advances. We rank sixteenth, or at least our women do. According to the World Health Organization, U.S. women live to 78.6 years on average. American men rank twenty-second, living on average to 71.6 years.

Many have observed, as well, that the senior years for many Americans are beset by disease, including osteoporosis, high blood pressure, heart disease, angina, and other chronic disorders, all of which destroy the quality of life. In other words, longevity is not the only marker for health, and it may not even be the best one.

People who live on diets dominated by grains and vegetables tend to have a much lower incidence of the major diseases, including the common cancers, heart disease, adult-onset diabetes, osteoporosis, and high blood pressure. The Chinese are a case in point. Cornell researchers found that the Chinese have extremely low rates of these illnesses—especially heart disease and the common cancers (breast, colon, and prostate)—as long as they subsist on their traditional diets of rice, vegetables, and small amounts of fish and other lean animal foods. However, when Chinese move to their own larger cities, or to the West, and adopt a more modern diet, their rates of disease go up to those that Americans typically experience.

After conducting the landmark study on the Chinese, Cornell researcher T. Colin Campbell stated, "We're basically a vegetarian species and should be eating a wide variety of plant foods and minimizing our intake of animal foods."

When we examine the human anatomy and physiology, we can see clearly that we were designed to eat a diet that was extremely rich in plant foods, plant nutrients, and fiber. The evidence for such a diet can begin with a look at our teeth, twenty of which are molars and premolars. These essentially

flat teeth are designed for grinding plant foods, but are inefficient for tearing flesh. Only four of our thirty-two teeth are
canine, unlike those of a dog's or cat's, which are clearly car-
nivorous. Unlike carnivores, we humans have a long digestive
tract, which is dependent for healthy function on fibrous
foods. Without adequate fiber, we are unable to eliminate
waste products and maintain healthy blood. Meat, when not
fully digested, often remains in the intestinal tract where it
can putrefy and cause disease, including tumors and colon
cancer.

Of all the constituents in the food supply, fat is clearly the
most toxic when eaten in excess. Fat elevates blood cholesterol, which in turn creates atherosclerotic plaques. The
plaques block blood and oxygen flow to cells and tissues.
Without adequate oxygen, cells die. When the inadequate
blood flow gets to the heart, a part of the heart can die, an
event called a heart attack; when the same conditions prevail
in the brain, a part of the brain can die, otherwise known as
a stroke. Both events can be lethal.

Fat also creates free radicals, or highly unstable molecules, which cause the decay of cells and organs. Free radicals cause the slow destruction of tissue. They are the
primary cause of aging, wrinkles, and more than sixty diseases, including heart disease, cancer, arthritis, Alzheimer's,
Parkinson's disease, and most of the other illnesses that kill
us.

Conversely, nutrients referred to as *anti*oxidants slow
down and sometimes even stop free-radical production, thus
slowing the aging process and preventing the development of
major diseases. Vegetables are the greatest sources of antioxidants, especially the vitamins C and E, and the vitamin A
precursor, beta-carotene. These and other antioxidants, such
as selenium, vitamin B_6, and glutathione, are found in abundance in whole grains, leafy greens, roots, squash, beans, and
sea vegetables.

Our primary biological need, once we reach adulthood, is

for energy. The body's primary source of energy is carbohydrates, found in whole grains, beans, vegetables, and fruit. These foods are also rich sources of vitamins, minerals, and chemicals that fight cancer.

Plant foods provide complex carbohydrates, which are slowly absorbed by the small intestine and therefore provide long-lasting energy and endurance. Simple sugars, on the other hand, provide a burst of energy that quickly burns off, often leaving people hypoglycemic, or anxious, fatigued, and weakened.

A diet composed of whole grains, fresh vegetables, beans, seaweed, fruit, and low-fat animal products meets all our nutritional needs. It promotes healthy circulation and optimizes the flow of blood and oxygen to cells; it boosts the immune system, and thus promotes healing; it slows the aging process; and it provides an abundance of complex carbohydrates, which in turn gives maximum energy. For all these reasons the diet I describe below provides the foundation for the restoration of good health.

Let's take a closer look at the main parts of the diet that humans were designed to eat. This is the kind of diet that I followed, which would be the same for most people living in a temperate climate. It was composed of fifty percent whole grains, such as brown rice, barley, millet, oats, and wheat; twenty-five to thirty percent vegetables, especially the green and leafy vegetables, such as collard, kale, mustard greens, and broccoli; ten percent beans and bean products, including chickpeas, lentils, *aduki* beans, tofu and tempeh; and the remainder composed of low-fat animal products, such as whitefish, and various soups, condiments, and fruit. The specific food groups are outlined next.

Whole Grains

When people began to sing songs about America, they sang about "amber waves of grain." When our ancestors considered all the foods available, they called grain "the staff of life." When the Chinese philosopher and sage Mencius ranked the most important aspects of any realm, he said the following: "The people are the most important element in the nation; the spirits of the land and grain are next." When the U.S. Department of Agriculture released its newest set of dietary guidelines for Americans, the food that scientists urged us to eat the most of was—grain—six to eleven servings per day!

Indeed, no matter how we approach food—from science, philosophy, traditional medicine, and culture, the one food that stands out as preeminent is whole grain. Why, we might ask, is such importance placed on this one food? Here's a short East–West answer to that question.

From the West

As I mentioned earlier, carbohydrates are our primary source of fuel. There are two types of carbohydrates—complex, which are long chains of sugar molecules; and simple, which are short and quickly metabolized sugars. Complex carbohydrates are broken down by saliva and enzymes in your intestines. These long chains of sugars are then made available to your bloodstream in a constant, methodical way, as if your body was feeding itself over several hours. Simple carbohydrates, which come in the form of white refined sugars, are absorbed into the bloodstream as soon as you put them into your mouth. Within minutes, they dramatically raise blood sugar levels and then quickly burn. They provide a quick burst of energy, but are quickly spent, leaving you without much available fuel. The result is that you feel tired, listless, moody, and anxious, a condition referred to as hypoglycemia.

Everyone wants to have energy, endurance, and stamina. Without energy there is no life. And clearly the best source of energy is from complex carbohydrates. The most abundant source of those are from whole grains. Whole grains—grains that have not been stripped of their nutrition by the refining process—provide the greatest assortment of nutrition in the food supply. Whole grains contain carbohydrates, protein, minerals, and vitamins, especially vitamin E and fiber. Animal foods contain lots of protein and fat, but no carbohydrates or fiber. Fruit contains lots of carbohydrates and fiber, but no protein.

Professor Paul C. Manglesdorf, a Harvard University agronomist, said, "A whole-grain cereal, if its food values are not destroyed by the overrefining of modern processing methods, comes closer than any other plant product to providing an adequate diet." No one, including Dr. Manglesdorf, is suggesting that we eat only whole grains, but when it comes to satisfying our overall needs for nutrition, grain is by far the most nutrient-rich food available.

Not only does it provide nutrition, but its fiber content also helps eliminate waste and fat. Fiber is indigestible matter. It swells with water inside the intestinal tract, making waste softer and peristalsis (the rhythmic contraction and expansion of the intestinal muscles) easier. All of these factors combine to make waste elimination easier and more frequent. Fiber also shrinks tumors in the intestines, and binds with fat and cholesterol to reduce blood cholesterol levels. From the health and scientific perspective alone, grain is a miraculous food.

From the East

Grain formed the basis of civilization among all peoples. But it also represented the basis of medicine, especially among Oriental peoples. In Chinese medicine, each grain was seen as an herb, having specific tonifying and strengthening effects on a specific set of organs. The chemistry of food was not understood by the Chinese, of course. They saw food from another view, as having specific energetic qualities. In Chinese medicine, a food's energetic nature is based upon how it grows, where it grows, and its structure or shape. Through centuries of study, the Chinese developed a system based upon how food affected individual parts of the body.

Here's a short list of whole grains, ways to use them, and individual health effects, according to Oriental medicine.

Brown Rice

Brown rice strengthens and boosts the function of the lungs and large intestine, according to Chinese medicine. It is the nature of brown rice—its underlying characteristic energy—that causes its life force, or *Qi,* to flow to these organs. In doing so, it is said to replenish the *Qi,* or life force, in both the lungs and large intestine. Brown rice also cleanses the large intestine, making its function more efficient and vital. The large intestine and lungs are seen as the places where the body stores its grief. By strengthening these organs, brown rice was also used to help eliminate, or let go of, longstanding grief from one's life. Brown rice is available as a short, medium, or long grain. (Short grain is consumed most frequently, but medium and long grain may be preferred during hot summer months.) Brown rice is prepared by pressure-cooking and boiling. It also can be combined with other grains, such as millet and barley, or with beans, such as *aduki* beans.

Barley

The organs that barley affects most are the kidneys and bladder. Barley, both its whole and lightly refined, or "pearled," form, stimulates and strengthens kidney and bladder function, according to Chinese medicine. It is especially recommended as a food in winter, when the Chinese maintain one's overall life force is focused more in these organs. Barley, both whole grain and "pearled," is delicious when cooked in a miso or tamari-shoyu broth. Barley is also wonderful in soups, stews, and cooked with a variety of other hearty vegetables and beans, such as carrots, onions, leeks, and shiitake mushrooms.

Wheat

The Chinese use wheat to help boost the function of the liver and gallbladder, to cleanse the organ, and to rebuild its *Qi*. The liver is seen as the place where we store our anger. Wheat helps the liver relax, to release pent-up tension and anger, and to restore equilibrium to the body and emotions. Wheat can be used in a variety of forms including: whole-wheat berries, bulgur; *fu* (baked puffed-wheat gluten), *seitan* (kneaded wheat gluten, meaty and hearty), whole-wheat bread, chapatis, and whole-wheat noodles.

Oats

Oats strengthen the liver and gallbladder. Whole, steel-cut, or rolled oats can be boiled as a breakfast cereal, and eaten plain or combined with a variety of fruits.

Corn

Corn strengthens the heart and small intestine, the places in the body in which joy is experienced and expressed, according to the Chinese. When the heart and small intestine functions are weak, joy is low and hysteria is more likely to occur. Corn is used to help strengthen these organs, as well as our capacity to experience more joy.

Buckwheat

Buckwheat is a hardy grass used as a grain, especially in winter because it has a warming effect on the body. It is said to strengthen the kidneys and bladder. Buckwheat can be used in the form of groats, noodles, and flour products, such as pancakes. It can also be cooked with sauerkraut and a variety of vegetables, including carrots and onions.

Amaranth

Amaranth strengthens the heart and small intestine.

Millet

Millet strengthens the spleen, pancreas, and stomach. The spleen is seen as the place where understanding resides in the body. People with weak spleens are either hard or cold, or overly solicitous to the point of being maudlin, say the Chinese healers. Millet strengthens the spleen and restores a balanced and understanding view of life. Millet can be boiled or pressure-cooked by itself, or cooked with a variety of vegetables, especially cauliflower and carrots, and other grains, such as barley or rice.

Sweet Rice

Like millet, sweet rice (a glutinous form of brown rice) boosts spleen function and assists the organ in healing itself. It also helps to strengthen the pancreas and stomach, and reestablishes biological function and emotional harmony. Sweet rice is used in making *mochi*, a kind of dumpling used in stews. Sometimes it is baked, which puffs the sweet rice up to become a kind of popover. *Mochi* is very hearty and strengthening. It's available in stores, prepackaged and ready to cook.

Noodles

Udon, whole-wheat pastas, *soba* (buckwheat), *jinenjo*—all
of these noodles are delicious in soups, broths, or sautéed
with vegetables. Noodle soup is rich in nutrition and provides
a wonderful way to include shiitake mushrooms in your diet.

Recommendations

I ate a grain dish two or three times per day and recommend it as the basis for almost every meal. Eat a wide variety
of grains. Pressure-cook grain, as well as boil. Pressure-cooking
locks in the nutrients and gives the grain a nuttier flavor.
Include noodles, especially in shiitake-and-tamari broth.

To Pressure Cook

For every 2 cups of brown rice, add 3½ to 4 cups of
water; add a pinch of sea salt; place lid on pot; turn on
high flame; bring to pressure (which takes about 10
minutes); once regulator jiggles intensely, turn down
flame to low and cook for 40 to 45 minutes. A stalk of
kombu seaweed can be used in place of sea salt occasionally.

Vegetables

"Boring" is the word most of us were trained to conjure up
every time we considered vegetables. But recent scientific
studies are putting vegetables in a whole new and exciting
light. Vegetables, scientists are finding, are powerful health
promoters that we simply cannot do without—that is, if we
want to maintain our health. Moreover, with just a little flair

and creativity, vegetables can be delicious foods. But let's concentrate on the health aspects for now. Here's an East–West guide to the exciting new world of the vegetable kingdom's healers.

From the West

Vegetables are your secret weapons against disease—lots of diseases, including cancer, heart disease, high blood pressure, cataracts, osteoporosis, and depressed immunity.

Cancer Fighters Extraordinaire

Broccoli, cabbage, kale, brussels sprouts, collard, and mustard greens contain a group of compounds, called indoles, which may prevent tumor-causing estrogen from targeting the breast. In animal studies they've been shown to switch on enzymes that prevent exposure to carcinogens. These vegetables also contain another cancer fighter, called sulforanphane. Sulforanphane has been called a "major and very potent" trigger for detoxifying tissues and blood, and for promoting production of cancer-preventive enzymes (*Proceedings of the National Academy of Sciences,* vol. 89, March 1992).

Other foods rich in phytochemicals and other cancer fighters are soybeans, citrus fruit, carrots, parsnips, celery, and parsley. "To harness anticarcinogenic activity, a combination of these vegetables would probably work best," says Herbert Pierson, PhD, cancer researcher, formerly of the National Cancer Institute. When researchers compared two groups of women—one with breast cancer and another group without the disease—they found that those who did not contract the illness ate significantly more vegetables, fruits, and fiber.

Researchers at the State University of New York compared the eating habits of 310 women with breast cancer to 316

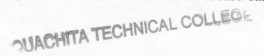

women free of the illness. The difference in their eating patterns, said the researchers, was that the women who did not get cancer ate diets richer in fiber, folic acid, carotenoids, and vitamin C—all derived from their increased intake of vegetables and fruit. The researchers theorized that the antioxidants, especially, provided protection against the disease.

Reduce Your Risk of Heart Disease

A study of 87,245 women done by Harvard Medical School showed that a single daily serving of fruits or vegetables rich in beta-carotene may reduce the risk of heart attack and stroke. "We found a twenty-two percent reduction in the risk of heart attack and a forty percent reduction in stroke for those women with high intakes of fruits and vegetables rich in beta-carotene compared to those with low intakes," says JoAnn E. Manson, M.D., project director for Brigham and Women's Hospital and Harvard Medical School. "We also found that high intakes of vitamin E [around 100 international units or more per day in supplement form] were associated with a thirty-six percent drop in heart attack risk."

Wondrous Sources of Calcium and other Minerals

In her book, *The Calcium Bible* (Warner Books, 1985), nutritionist Patricia Hausman, MS, shows that green vegetables rank with dairy products as great sources of calcium—without the fat, lactose, purines, antibiotics, and steroids that most milk products contain. Here's a short list of greens:

- 1 cup of cooked collard greens: 360 mg. of calcium

- 1 cup of fresh cooked broccoli: 140 mg.

- 1 cup of cooked bok choy: 250 mg.

- 1 cup of cooked kale: 210 mg.

- 1 cup of cooked turnip greens: 200 mg.

- 1 cup of cooked mustard greens: 190 mg.

Vegetables also contain iron, magnesium, zinc, potassium, manganese, and selenium—minerals that scientists tell us strengthen the immune system and are essential to healthy metabolism.

Great Sources of Vitamin C

Most people don't realize that some of the best sources of vitamin C are vegetables, especially broccoli, cabbage, cauliflower, bell peppers, and squash. Broccoli and bell peppers, to name just two, contain richer quantities of vitamin C than citrus fruits. Here are some of the numbers, according to the U.S. Department of Agriculture:

- Broccoli: 98 mg. per cooked cup

- Brussels sprouts: 97 mg. per cooked cup

- Orange juice: 97 mg. per 8-oz. serving

- Green pepper: whole, 95 mg.

- Strawberries: 85 mg. per cup

- Cauliflower: 69 mg. per cooked cup

Fiber

Fiber maintains the health of your digestive tract, especially your colon. An abundance of scientific research has shown that those who eat diets rich in fiber have far lower rates of colon and breast cancers than those who abstain from fibrous foods. Vegetables, grains, and fruit are the only sources of fiber available to use. Animal foods contain no fiber.

Gold Mines of Antioxidants

Vegetables are rich sources of beta-carotene and vitamins C and E, all antioxidants and powerful immune boosters and disease fighters. Squash, broccoli, collards, kale, mustard greens, brussels sprouts, carrots, parsnips, and other yellow vegetables are the sources of beta-carotene. Whole grains, vegetables, and vegetable oils contain vitamin E.

From the East

The Oriental healer sees the vegetable kingdom with the right brain, so to speak. He or she views it as a living whole, shaped by energies that are implicit within the vegetable and thus make it grow according to its unique nature. A leafy green, for example, fans upward and outward because its energies captured within the vegetable cause it to grow in this way. A grain, on the other hand, is tight and compact because the energies are turning inward, like an ever-tightening spiral. A root grows downward into the earth, like a pointy spiral, similar to a corkscrew. All of these ways of development suggest how the food will react within your body. The Chinese worked out an elaborate system in which each food was seen as having specific energetic properties and thus made it an herb, or a poison, for specific organs. Here's a short overview of vegetables and their herbal effects.

The following vegetables and grains are considered healing foods. Eat at least one serving of each column per day.

Leafy Greens	*Round and Ground*	*Roots*
Asparagus	Artichokes	Burdock
Beet Greens	Bamboo Shoots	Carrot
Carrot Tops	Beets	Celery
Chinese Cabbage	Broccoli	Chicory Root
Collard Greens	Brussels Sprouts	Daikon Radish
Curly Dock	Cabbage	Dandelion Root
Daikon Radish	Cucumber	*Jinenjo* Potato
Green Peas	Icicle Radish	Lotus Root
Dandelion Greens	Leeks	Parsnip
Endive	Shiitake Mushrooms	Red Radish
Escarole	Okra	Rutabaga
Kale	Squash	Salsify Root
Kohlrabi	Acorn Squash	Turnip
Lamb's Quarters	Butternut Squash	
Leek Greens	*Hakkaido* Pumpkin	
Lettuce	Hubbard Squash	
Mustard Greens	Pumpkin	
Parsley	Yellow Squash	
Plantain	Zucchini	
Scallion	Snow Peas	
Shepherd's Purse	String Beans	
Sorrel	Sweet Potatoes	
Sprouts	Yams	
Swiss Chard	Onions	
Turnip Greens		
Watercress		

Cooking Vegetables

- Steaming—3 to 5 minutes, depending on the size and consistency, in a ½ inch of water.

- Boiling—Boil in water with a couple drops of tamari or shoyu (optional) for 3 to 5 minutes. Nutrients are lost in greater quantities when vegetables are boiled in a larger volume of water over a longer period of time. Reuse vegetable broth in soups and sauces to add nutrients.

- Sautéing—Sauté with oils (preferably olive or sesame). Coat frying pan lightly, add washed and cut vegetables, and sauté for about 5 minutes.

- Baking—The best way to prepare squashes. Cut squash, bake at 375° to 400° F for 1 to 2 hours until tender. Summer squash and zucchini require far less time—20 to 35 minutes depending on size. Yams and sweet potatoes require higher heat, between 400° and 500° F for about 1 hour.

Beans

Let's face it: Many people avoid beans because they have a reputation for causing flatulence. But that occurs only in those who eat beans sporadically, don't chew them well, don't soak them before cooking, and do not cook them in *kombu* seaweed, which alkalizes the beans and helps to make them more digestible. Beans are far less gas-producing for those who eat them regularly, soak them, and cook them with *kombu.* In any case, people who avoid beans because of their unsociable effects are missing out on one of the most delicious, nutritious, and revitalizing foods available to us.

Here's an East–West guide to the nutritious and health-protecting properties of beans.

From the West

Beans are the greatest source of protein in the vegetable kingdom. Collectively known as legumes, beans and peas generally contain between twenty and thirty percent protein.

They are also rich sources of complex carbohydrates and fiber, and contain significant amounts of vitamins and minerals. One hundred grams of soybeans, for example, contain 226 mg. of calcium; 554 mg. of phosphorus; 8.4 mg. of iron; and 1,677 mg. of potassium, according to the U.S. Department of Agriculture (USDA). One hundred grams of *aduki* beans contain 21 mg. of protein. A hundred grams of chickpeas contain 20 mg. of protein, and whole lentils contain 25 mg. of protein, according to USDA. All beans contain A and B vitamins, as well.

As with grains, beans contain soluble fibers, which bind with fat and cholesterol, and lower blood cholesterol levels. This prevents atherosclerosis, or cholesterol plaque, that forms in the arteries to the heart and brain and causes heart attack and stroke. But beans have other properties that scientists are just beginning to appreciate. The American Health Foundation reported that beans may well be the reason Hispanic women suffer such low rates of breast cancer. Hispanic women, who experience far lower rates of breast cancer than white women, eat twice as many beans, the scientists found. Upon further study, the researchers discovered that beans contain high amounts of an estrogen-blocking chemical, phytoestrogens, which may protect against breast disease, including malignancies of the breast.

All soybeans and soybean products—including tofu, tempeh, *natto,* tamari, and miso—contain "genistein," a substance that blocks blood vessels from attaching to cancer cells and tumors, thus preventing cancer cells from getting oxygen and nutrition (*Proceedings of the National Academy of Sciences,* vol. 90, April 1993).

Western science has demonstrated that excesses of protein, especially from animal sources, weaken bones and kidneys, and leads to osteoporosis. Once inside the body, excess protein is converted to ammonia and then to uric acid. That acid, which must be removed from the bloodstream by the kidneys, can weaken kidney function and even destroy kidney tissue. The body responds to this excess acid by releasing calcium from bones. Calcium is highly alkaline, and thus neutralizes the acid produced by protein. This, of course, weakens the bones and leads to osteoporosis.

Animal protein has also been linked to various forms of cancer, including those of the prostate, colon, and breast. Beans provide low to moderate amounts of protein, ideal for kidneys and the health of bones. It is for this reason that the U.S. surgeon general and other leading scientists are encouraging people to get more of their protein from vegetable sources, such as beans, than from animal sources.

In the late 1960s and early 1970s, Frances Moore Lappe popularized the notion that beans contain only some of the eight essential amino acids, or the building blocks of protein. She helped foster the idea that beans had to be combined with grains or seeds to provide a "complete" protein. This belief was based on the research of Osborn and Mendel, who in 1914 studied the protein requirements of rats and automatically assumed they were identical to humans. However, in 1952 William Rose proved that most individual natural foods contain all the amino acids, including the eight essential amino acids, as long as the food was not stripped of its original nutrition by refining. Beans, like other whole foods, are excellent sources of complete protein. In fact, scientists have pointed out that people have met their protein requirements and lived healthfully for extended periods of time on potatoes and water alone.

From the East

In Chinese medicine beans are revered for their tonifying and strengthening effects on the kidneys and bladder. Small but daily consumption of beans is used to treat and strengthen the kidneys and bladder. All beans are helpful to the kidneys and bladder, but kidney beans, *azuki,* chickpeas, lentils, soybeans, and black beans are regarded as especially healing.

The Chinese see the kidney as providing *Qi,* or life force, to the sex organs. All such disorders, including sexual dysfunction, menstrual or ovarian diseases, and prostate or testicular disorders, are treated, in part, by healing the kidneys.

The kidneys are highly sensitive to excesses of fat and sodium. Fat causes cholesterol plaques to clog the tiny nephrons, or the basic filtering unit within the organs. This can destroy the kidneys. Sodium has a paradoxical relationship with the kidneys. Small to moderate amounts actually tonify and strengthen kidney function, according to Chinese medicine. But excesses cause too much contraction of the organs, thus preventing them from filtering waste from the body. This excessive contraction of the kidneys has the same effect as pinching a hose while water is running: pressure builds behind the pinch, resulting in high blood pressure.

Beans are said to be warming foods, meaning that they stimulate circulation and thus warm the body. They also contain moderate amounts of monounsaturated and polyunsaturated fats, which lower cholesterol somewhat and thus assist in the elimination of fat from the kidneys. These fats make beans a rich and luscious food. Like Western physicians, Oriental healers see beans as acid-producing foods, because of their protein content. Interestingly, Chinese healers have maintained for thousands of years that the *Qi* emanating from the kidneys nourishes and maintains the bones. Thus, like Western doctors, the Chinese recognized the relationship between kidneys and bones.

A fundamental principle in all traditional medicine is the need for balance and moderation in all things, including the consumption of beans. Too many beans, and too much protein, create too much acid and can be harmful to health. Most Oriental healers recommend that small amounts of beans—about a cup—be eaten once a day.

In addition to the standard beans are tofu—a moderately refined soybean product that is rich in calcium and protein—and tempeh, a fermented soybean food that is rich in digestive enzymes. Finally, there is *natto,* a fermented soybean condiment used on rice and other grains, and sometimes in soups. All fermented soybean foods assist in digestion by providing friendly bacteria that helps make nutrients more available to the small intestine.

Recommendations

- Eat beans five to seven times per week. Choose any of the common beans, especially *aduki,* black turtle, chickpeas, kidney beans, navy, split peas, and soybeans.

- Eat fermented soybean products, such as tempeh, *natto,* miso, tamari (a condiment used in cooking, very like soy sauce), and shoyu (also like soy sauce).

- Cook beans with a piece of *kombu* seaweed; add seaweed at the start of cooking. (Do not add salt until beans are 80 percent done.)

- Eat tofu occasionally. Once a week sauté tempeh in sesame or olive oil.

Cooking Beans

- Boiling—This is the preferred method for cooking most beans. Soak beans overnight and boil them with a single stalk of *kombu* seaweed, which will cause the beans to be more digestible. Add a pinch of sea salt or a few drops of tamari or shoyu when the beans are 80 percent done. Boil for about 1½ hours to 2 hours.

- Pressure-cooking—(Be sure that pressure-cooker regulator is clear and clean before pressure-cooking beans because beans can clog the regulator.) Add 3 cups of water per cup of beans; cook with a stalk of *kombu* seaweed. Cover pressure cooker, lock shut, bring to pressure, as indicated by the hissing of the regulator (usually requires approximately 10 minutes), reduce heat to low, and cook for 45 minutes.

- Baking—Place beans in pot of water; 3 to 4 cups of water per cup of beans; add stalk of *kombu* seaweed, if desired, and a pinch of sea salt. Bake at 350° F for 3 to 4 hours. When beans are 80 percent done, add a variety of condiments or spices, such as raisins, miso, tamari, shoyu, others.

- Tempeh and tofu, can be sautéed, baked, steamed and boiled; they can be added to soups and stews. Tofu and *natto* can be eaten raw.

Seaweeds

Like the ocean itself, sea vegetables possess a vast supply of vitamins and minerals essential for life. Not only do they contain great quantities of individual nutrients, but they also possess a wide variety. The benefits of sea vegetables go beyond nutrition, however, as this East–West guide to sea vegetables reveals.

From the West

No other food on earth packs as much nutrition into such tiny volumes as sea vegetables. One hundred grams of *hijiki* seaweed contains 1,400 mg. of calcium, according to the U.S. Department of Agriculture and the Food Composition Table of East Asia. The same size serving of milk contains 118 mg. The recommended daily allowance (RDA) for calcium is 800 to 1,000 mg. That's one of the amazing aspects of sea vegetables: Even small amounts of these foods often come close to, or exceed, the RDA.

Nori seaweed, which can be purchased as "sushi nori," requires no cooking. It comes in flat sheets and can be used to wrap around rice or noodles to make sushi, or ground up and sprinkled on grain. One hundred grams of nori contains 28.3 mg. of iron (the RDA is 15 mg. per day); 3,503 mg. of potassium (the RDA is 1,800); 17,800 International Units (IU) of beta-carotene (the vegetable source of vitamin A; the RDA is 4,500 mg.); 1.34 mg. of riboflavin B_2 (the RDA is 1.7 mg.); and 22.2 mg. of protein (the RDA is 65 mg.). At the same time, sea vegetables contain only small amounts of fat. One hundred grams of nori, for example, contains 1.1 g. of fat, as compared to whole milk, which contains 3.5 g. of fat, or a hundred grams of egg, which contain 11.5 g. of fat.

In fact, sea vegetables are rich sources of calcium, iron, beta-carotene, vitamins E and K, and the B vitamins (thiamine, riboflavin, and niacin). They even contain B_{12}. Many are good sources of vitamin C. Nori, for example, contains 14 mg. of C; *wakame,* a leafy seaweed often used in soups and stews, contains 15 mg. of vitamin C. Sea vegetables also have substantial amounts of fiber.

Many people wonder whether or not sea vegetables contain pollutants, since parts of the ocean are polluted themselves. But Maine Coast Sea Vegetables, one of many sea vegetable harvesters who conduct regular tests on the seaweeds they harvest, have found no traces of PCBs, hydrocarbons, and pesticides in their sea vegetables. Independent authorities, such as the Maine Department of Natural Resources, confirm that the sea vegetables are safe.

"Nobody has shown that seaweeds accumulate anything toxic to any appreciable level," Dr. Mark Littler, botanist at the Smithsonian's Museum of Natural History in Washington, DC, told *The New York Times*.

Another concern some people have is the sodium content of sea vegetables. By weight, sea vegetables do contain significant amounts of sodium, but nutritionists point out that the sodium can be reduced by rinsing and soaking the seaweeds before cooking. Also, seaweeds contain substantial amounts of potassium, the balancing electrolyte that helps to maintain the body's fluid balance. *The New York Times* reported that the sodium–potassium balance in seaweeds is three parts sodium to one part potassium, very similar to the body's ratio of five parts sodium to one part potassium. Table salt, the greatest source of sodium for most people, has a ratio of ten thousand parts sodium to one part potassium—clearly the greater threat to human health. Finally, nutritionists point out that even those who eat lots of sea vegetables do not consume them in great quantities at any one meal. Rather, they are eaten in small amounts, which provide an abundance of nutrition, but limited amounts of sodium.

Researchers at McGill University in Montreal, Canada, have found that sodium alginate, found in many seaweeds, protects bones from absorbing radioactive particles and heavy metals. Indeed, sea vegetables—long seen by scientists as an important source of nutrition in the world's future—are among the most important foods we can eat today.

From the East

For the Oriental healer, sea vegetables are a medicinal food that can be eaten daily. The organs they affect the most are the kidneys and bladder, or what Chinese refer to as the

Water Element. Sea vegetables cause the kidneys and bladder to collect or gather energy, or life force, making them more vital and efficient. Seaweeds are said to tonify the kidneys and bladder by causing them to contract slightly.

Seaweeds help to cleanse the kidneys and bladder of accumulated waste. They also support the body's efforts at protecting the organs and rebuilding their *Qi,* or life force. Such foods as coffee, sugar, and spices have the opposite effect on the kidneys; they scatter energy and expand the kidneys and bladder. In the process the organs become weak, lethargic, and inefficient. Toxins are therefore able to accumulate within the organs and cause their decline.

The kidneys are seen in Chinese medicine as the place where the human will is housed. People with strong will are said to have strong kidneys. Oriental healers encourage people to eat regular amounts of seaweeds to maintain the strength of their will. If the will is weak, the kidneys must be treated, in part with regular consumption of seaweed.

The kidneys are also the organs that provide the body with its underlying vitality and enduring strength. The Chinese maintain that the kidneys distribute *Qi,* or life force, throughout the body. They are the organs that give us the power to fight difficulties with courage and stamina. Like the sea itself, sea vegetables are restorative for mind, body, and spirit.

Common sea vegetables

- *Arame*—This is commonly used as a vegetable itself—cooked with other vegetables, such as carrots, and sprinkled with lemon and sesame seeds—or it's used in soups and stews. Rich in protein, carbohydrates, vitamins A and B, minerals, including calcium. Cook for 30 minutes with carrots, onions, lemon juice, alone or in soups and stews.

- *Dulse*—It can be eaten raw, roasted and added to rice and other grains as a condiment, or marinated in lemon juice, or added to soups and stews. Rich in iron (32 mg./100 g. serving), potassium, beta-carotene, and vitamins A, E, B, and C, protein, iodine, minerals, and trace elements.

- *Hijiki*—It can be eaten as a vegetable itself, or added to soups and stews. Loaded with protein, vitamins A and B, calcium, phosphorus, iron, and many trace elements, *hijiki* provides 29 mg. of iron per 100 g. serving. Boil with carrots, onions, daikon radish for 1 hour to 1½ hours.

- *Kombu*—Rich in calcium (955 mg./100 g. serving), *Kombu* can be added when boiling beans to make beans more digestible. Cooked also as a vegetable with carrots, onions, rutabagas, turnips, and daikon.

- *Nori* and *Sushi Nori*—Perhaps the easiest sea vegetable to use, and the one most acceptable to the novice palate, is nori. Nori comes in sheets and is used to make nori rolls, sushi, and rice balls (brown rice covered with nori). Roast nori over an open flame for 5 seconds; when it turns bright green, remove from flame. Nori can also be crumbled into a condiment. Rich in vitamins A, B family, C, and D, calcium, phosphorus, iron, and trace elements. Very versatile, and highly nutritious. Sushi nori is pre-roasted nori that requires no preparation. Just take it out of the package and use as desired.

- *Wakame*—Here is a leafy, rich sea vegetable that is used mostly in soups (miso soup) and stews. Cooks in 20 minutes. Rich in protein, calcium (1,300 mg./100 g. serving), iron, potassium, beta-carotene, B vitamins, and vitamin C. Very nutritious.

Recommendations

- Eat sea vegetables five to seven times per week.

- Eat only one to two tablespoon-size portions per serving.

- Rinse and soak seaweeds thoroughly before using to remove excess sodium.

- Eat sushi nori seaweed to adjust to flavor of seaweed. Sushi nori does not require any preparation; simply remove from package, wrap rice or other grains in the seaweed, and eat like a sandwich.

- Nori is a wonderful seaweed to start children on.

Miso Soup

Miso is a soybean paste that has been fermented in salt anywhere from two months to two years. Often a grain is added to the mix, such as wheat, brown rice, barley, or millet. Miso was created by the Japanese and used traditionally as a base for soups, stews, and sauces. A staple in Japan for countless generations, miso soup is regarded as a powerful healing food. Over the centuries, a whole folklore has sprung up around miso soup. "Miso strengthens the weak and softens the hard," goes one traditional saying. The meaning is that it tonifies and restores the vitality to organs that are sick and lethargic, while it softens and breaks up stagnation, cysts, and tumors. Of course, Western scientists and physicians had little interest in such traditional foods, and their medicinal uses—that is, until recently, when science began to show that the folklore may well be true.

From the West

In April 1993 it was reported (*Proceedings of the National Academy of Sciences,* vol. 90, pp. 2690–2994) that scientists had isolated a substance in miso that effectively blocks blood flow to tumors, thus starving them of the essentials of life. The scientists called the substance "genistein." It blocks blood vessels from attaching to tumors, a process known as angiogenesis. Cancer cells and tumors, like all other cells and tissues in the body, need oxygen and nutrition to survive. In order for them to get both, they need blood. Thus, cancer is sustained within the body by blood vessels that grow to the cells and support their life. The genistein in miso soup blocks blood vessels from attaching to the cancer cells, and thus literally suffocates and starves the tumor.

In reporting the findings, *The New York Times* (April 13, 1993) stated the following: "That talent could have significant implications for both the prevention and treatment of many types of solid tumors, including malignancies of the breast, prostate and brain."

Dr. Judah Folkmann of the Harvard Medical School, who has studied how blood vessels form to support the growth of cancerous tumors, said that genistein may be an ideal form of cancer therapy, one that attacks the cancer cells but leaves normal cells unaffected.

The National Academy of Sciences report comes after numerous studies by the Japanese National Cancer Center showing that populations of people who eat miso soup regularly have thirty-three percent fewer incidences of cancer than those who never eat it. In addition, miso is rich in friendly bacteria, such as lactobacilli, which aids digestion and makes nutrients more available to the small intestine, and is also a good source of protein.

From the East

In fact, one of the most celebrated reports of miso's protective effects came from Japanese physician Tatsuichiro Akizuki, M.D., who used miso to treat the sick and wounded who had survived the dropping of the atomic bomb upon Nagasaki. He recorded his experience as follows:

"On August 9, 1945, the atomic bomb was dropped on Nagasaki. It killed many thousands of people. The hospital I was in charge of at the time was located only one mile from the center of the blast. It was destroyed completely. My assistants and I helped many victims who suffered from the effects of the bomb. In my hospital there was a large stock of miso and tamari [the liquid that comes off the miso during the fermentation process and is used as a condiment and soup stock]. We also kept plenty of brown rice and *wakame* [sea vegetable]. So I fed my coworkers brown rice and miso soup. I remember that none of them suffered from the atomic radiation. I believe this is because they had been eating miso soup."

Miso is highly alkaline and has long been used to treat stomach and digestive problems. Its natural alkalinity balances stomach and bile acids, which accumulate in the duodenum, the first part of the small intestine. These acids are among the causes of most ulcers. Miso alkalizes the entire digestive tract, thus protecting the life of delicate cells and tissues that exist throughout the small and large intestines. All traditional cultures prize fermented foods, such as pickles, sauerkraut, and beer. Miso is perhaps the most highly revered fermented food in Japan; others include tamari (the liquid that comes off miso), shoyu (Japanese soy sauce), tempeh (fermented soybean patties), *natto* (fermented soybean condiment), and sake (or rice wine). All of these foods offer friendly bacteria that assists in digestion. This bacteria also produces oxygen, which further enriches the health and vitality of the intestinal tract.

Traditionally, miso is seen as particularly strengthening to the spleen, large intestine, and kidneys. The spleen thrives under alkaline conditions, according to the Chinese, but is harmed by acidic foods, such as sweet wines, sugar, and strong spices. Miso alkalizes and strengthens the spleen. The spleen, in turn, passes *Qi,* or life force, to the large intestine; in this way, it boosts large intestine function. Many people who suffer from digestive disorders are actually suffering from spleen imbalance, according to Chinese medicine. Miso also boosts the large intestine function by alkalizing the organ's environment and enriching it with friendly bacteria. Finally, it tightens and tonifies the kidneys, making the organs more fit and vital. For all of these reasons, miso is a wondrous food. There are many types of miso available today. Among the most popular are rice, millet, barley, and chickpea misos.

Recommendations

- Eat miso soup five to seven times per week.

- Use ¼ to ½ teaspoon of miso per cup of soup

- Vary your misos: Use barley, rice, chickpea and other light misos regularly.

Miso Soup Recipe

Miso soup begins by adding *wakame* seaweed to boiling water. Simmer. Cut vegetables such as carrots or onions while the seaweed cooks (about a minute). Add vegetables and cook until they are soft—usually about 20 minutes. Reduce flame to low. Add miso to broth, cook for a few minutes, and then serve hot.

Animal Foods

- Whitefish and salmon are the preferred animal foods. Among the most common and nutritious whitefish are cod, scrod, haddock, flounder, halibut, and sole.

- Whitefish and salmon have omega polyunsaturated oils, which lower cholesterol level.

- Minimize or eliminate all red meat, dairy food, and eggs.

- Minimize or eliminate poultry. If you continue to eat poultry, try to eat only small amounts of organically grown chicken and turkey, and use it sparingly in soups. The white meat of poultry is lower in fat than the dark. Avoid the skin of poultry, which is rich in fat.

Condiments and Dressings

- Roasted sesame seeds—Roast sesame seeds in a dry frying pan. Roast *kombu* seaweed in oven. Grind roasted sesame seeds with roasted *kombu* and add to grain as a condiment. (You may soak sesame seeds for a few hours or overnight and throw away water to eliminate oxalic acid, which binds with the calcium and makes it inaccessible to the body.)
- Roasted black sesame seeds—Roast in dry frying pan. Add *shiso* leaves or sea salt. For *shiso* leaves, the ratio should be 10 parts sesame seeds to 1 part *shiso* leaves; for sea salt, the ratio should be 17 to 1.
- Roasted small fish, ground into flakes, e.g., small dried sardines (called *chirimen iriko*) can be purchased in an Oriental food store.

Rich in iron, vitamin D, calcium, and other nutrients:

- Rice vinegar

- Tofu-based salad dressings, if health permits

- *Umeboshi* dressings

- *Mirin*

- Grated gingerroot

- Lemon juice, sliced lemons, as on fish

- Horseradish

- Scallions, chives, parsley

- Natural shoyu and tamari

- Miso-based dressings, add *kuzu* to thicken

- Sauerkraut

- Lemon water

- Roasted sunflower seeds

Oils

Oil is liquid fat. Vegetable oils—referred to as polyunsaturated and monounsaturated fats—lower blood cholesterol levels somewhat, but excessive use of vegetable oils has been linked to cancer.

Oils should be minimized. Sauté once or twice a week. Do

not fry. If you are using diet as an adjunct to medical therapy, avoid oil as much as possible to maximize circulation, reduce weight, and prevent disease. Corn, sesame, and olive oils are less harmful and preferred.

Snacks and Desserts

Use unrefined, natural foods as snacks. Avoid oily, sugared, or processed foods. Use whole grains as snacks for their fiber, vitamin, and mineral content.

- Fruit

- Cooked fruit

- Rice cakes

- Dried fruit in season

- Popcorn

- Puffed grains

- Seeds and nuts (small amounts, if health permits)

- Natural candies made without sugar, such as yinnies, barley malt candy, etc.

- Good-quality whole-grain bread, preferably sourdough. Steam bread before eating to make it more digestible. Avoid yeasted bread.

- Natural, unsweetened apple butters, jams, and other spreads. Avoid sugar, fat, and chemical additives in all jams and spreads.

Drinks and Beverages

In general, drink when thirsty. However, people with cold and/or dry conditions often neglect their thirst, or are unconscious of the need for liquids. One of the ways we can become aware of our thirst is to be conscious whenever we drink pure spring water. How does your body react when you drink? Do you suddenly become aware that you were thirsty all along? Does your body respond to the water by sending signals of gratitude for drinking? Do you automatically know that you do not need water and therefore cease to drink? Reflect on your body's reaction whenever you drink and control your intake of liquids accordingly.

- Drink spring water; *kukicha* twig tea; noncaffeinated grain coffee, such as pero; mild herbal teas, such as chamomile, ginger tea, lemon tea, mu tea

- Avoid spicy and highly aromatic teas

Herbal Remedies for Healing

One of the ways I maintain my health today is by eating foods and taking herbal remedies that either support general health, or are particularly useful when I catch a cold. Today scientists are discovering that the herbs and healing foods used by our ancestors and traditional healers for generations are indeed powerful and effective at treating illness and keeping us healthy. Below is a guide to herbs and healing foods that can be used to assist in healing specific conditions or protect against disease. All of these herbs and foods are widely available in natural foods stores, health food stores, and many supermarkets.

If any condition persists, be sure to consult a physician or health practitioner. But for mild or chronic problems that persist in spite of medicine, try the herbs and foods described below.

Aloe Vera (Juice or Gel)

Used to treat skin problems, especially cuts, abrasions, wounds, and burns, aloe vera prevents scarring and encourages healing. The gel can be drawn directly from the pulpy aloe vera plant leaves. Apply the fresh juice or gel directly to the affected area. This herb has been used since the ancient Egyptians. It is safe, highly effective, and increasingly turns up in products from skin lotions to shampoos.

Burdock Root

Used to promote the health and function of the kidneys, lungs, and liver, it is also used to treat chronic skin problems. It can be taken as a tea—boil 1 teaspoon (tsp.) of dried herb in 1 cup of water for 10 minutes; steep for 10 more minutes; drink twice a day for one week. Or used as a tincture (drops). Use 10 to 30 drops in water; twice a day, for one week. Do not take herb longer than a week. Combine with dandelion and *echinacea* (see listings for *Echinacea* and Dandelion herbs) for strong immune booster and antifungal treatment.

Burdock can be found in most of our backyards. It's free for the taking and a wonderful promoter of health. It can be dried at home and chopped up to be used as an herbal tea (formula described above). Use burdock for skin problems and as a tonifier and promoter of kidney function.

Calendula

Used to treat skin problems, especially pimples and acne, it is antiseptic and anti-inflammatory. It heals and soothes. It is often found as part of an herbal salve. Apply directly to skin. Can be purchased as a dried herb, boiled, and used in a compress on the skin.

Cascara Sagrada

This can be one of the most effective and powerful laxatives available. Use 15 to 30 drops of a tincture in a small amount of water, three times per day, once in the morning, once at midday, and once before bed. Use 10 to 15 drops for children. Do not use more than four days straight. The herb is best used for short periods. It can create a dependency or lose its potency after a time.

Chamomile

Used to treat skin problems, it soothes the skin and makes it smooth. It's often part of an herbal salve. The common herb tea speeds up a process called phagocytosis, or the proliferation of phagocyte cells, according to Dr. James Duke, a botanist and expert on herbs at the U.S. Department of Agriculture. The tea, which comes in tea bags and is commonly found in stores, also relaxes, makes sleep deeper and more restful, and helps relieve insomnia.

Cinnamon

Dr. James Duke has found that cinnamon increases the number of certain immune cells, called leukocytes. Research at the HNRC at Tufts has found that cinnamon triples insulin's ability to metabolize glucose, or blood sugar. By increasing the efficiency of insulin, cinnamon protects against diabetes and lowers hunger and sugar cravings, thus making it easier to control weight.

Clay

Usually bought as French Green clay, but other clays are often just as good if French Green can not be found. To treat a boil or pimple: Mix a tablespoon or more of the clay-powder with just enough water to cause the powder to become a clay (usually it requires no more than a few tablespoons of water). Apply to the skin and let it dry. The clay can be applied in the morning and at night, until the boil or pimple has opened and drained, after which apply Tea Tree Oil or herbal balm to promote healing. Clay, such as French Green clay, can be purchased in most health and natural foods stores.

Cumin

Israeli scientists have found that people who regularly add cumin to their food have lower rates of urinary tract cancers, including those of the bladder and prostate. (See also Saw Palmetto for prostate.) Scientists in India confirmed these findings and discovered that cumin greatly increased the body's production of a detoxifying agent, called GST, which is known to have strong cancer-inhibiting properties.

Dandelion

Used traditionally to strengthen liver, spleen, and heart, dandelion promotes blood-cleansing functions of liver, and lymph movement and drainage. It is also given to people suffering from hepatitis to promote flow of bile from the liver. Eaten as a vegetable in springtime, especially. Dried herb can be taken as tea (1 tbs. of herb per 1 cup of water; boil for 10 minutes; steep for 10 minutes; drink daily for three days to a week). Can be taken as a tincture: 10 to 30 drops in cup of water, three to five times per week, for four weeks.

The leaves of dandelions are common everywhere in North America. Harvest them before the plant flowers, however.

After flowering, the plant becomes highly bitter and loses much of its vitality and healing effect.

Echinacea

Among the most widely used herbs in the world to treat infections and symptoms of colds and flu, it is increasingly used by doctors as a replacement for antibiotics. One of the most powerful and effective immune boosters and antibiotics in the plant kingdom. Promotes healing. Herbalist Michael Tierra, author of *Planetary Herbology* (Lotus Press, 1988), says that "*echinacea* stimulates the body's immune system against all infections and inflammatory conditions, counteracts pus, and stimulates digestion. . . . *Echinacea* is one of the most powerful and effective remedies against all kinds of bacterial and viral infections."

Use fifteen to thirty drops of the tincture in water, three to five times per day until condition improves. A child's dose is usually one half the adult dosage, or 15 drops, two times per day. Do not use for more than five days to a week. Though there are no harmful side effects, it can reduce intestinal flora and constipate.

The dried *echinacea* herb can be boiled in water to make a tea. You can combine *echinacea* with dandelion and burdock (also dried herbs), to create an immune-boosting tea. Boil 1 tbs. of each herb in 3 cups of water for 10 minutes. Let steep for 15 minutes and drink.

Eucalyptus

Eucalyptus is used as an inhalation against colds and flu; to promote circulation in lungs, break up congestion, and improve breathing. Often combined with pine needle, cloves, and thyme. Place the herbs in a vaporizer, along with water. Use leaves or oil of leaves. Hold towel over head to create a tent over herbal steam and vaporizer. Inhale three times per day for 10 minutes. This also can be left on in your room at night to help breathing. Herbs can be added to pot of boiling water if vaporizer is not available.

Garlic

According to Michael Wargovich, M.D., professor of medicine at M.D. Anderson Cancer Center in Houston, Texas, garlic is highly anti-cancer and promotes health in a wide variety of ways. Garlic causes the liver to metabolize and neutralize carcinogens that would otherwise produce cancer cells and tumors. According to Dr. Wargovich, garlic stimulates the liver to more effectively identify these poisons and turn them into harmless, water-soluble compounds. Garlic also encourages a variety of detoxifying enzymes to be produced by the body, some of which directly attack cancer cells and tumors. Studies have found that the rates of stomach and colorectal cancers are lower among those who have high garlic consumption. Scientists speculate that garlic may block the tumor-promoting effects of a certain group of fatty acids called prostaglandins, which are hormonelike substances in the body. Prostaglandins may encourage tumor growth when they go unregulated.

Researchers at the National Cancer Institute say that garlic also has health-promoting effects when eaten cooked, as well. Consequently, scientists are recommending that garlic be used both raw and cooked.

Gingerroot

Usually used as a tea or fresh grated as a condiment, ginger tea promotes circulation; improves digestion; and is good for motion sickness, indigestion, or other stomach problems. Ginger tea also promotes stronger menses and helps to reduce symptoms of PMS. To make gingerroot tea: grate 1 tbs. of fresh ginger, place in bottom of a cup and then pour hot water over. Add 1 or 2 drops of tamari. (Instead of hot water, use a mild tea, such as *kukicha* tea, which is alkaline, non-aromatic, and contains minerals. It can be found in your natural foods store.)

Goldenseal

One of the most universally recognized herbal healers in the plant kingdom, goldenseal is antibacterial, anti-inflammatory, astringent, immune boosting, and promotes healing. When used externally, it treats wounds (as part of an herbal salve), abrasions, skin irritations, and hemorrhoids (also as a suppository). It is effective against all types of skin problems, including vaginal yeast infections.

Internally, promotes the body's blood-cleansing functions, reduces inflammation, treats infection, boosts immune function, regulates menses, reduces bleeding, shrinks blood vessels. Can be combined with water and used as an eyewash. Herbalists recommend 15 to 30 drops in water, two or three times per day. After ten days, it can reduce intestinal flora and cause constipation. It can also be used to treat sore throats. Apply tincture drops to a cotton swab and daub back of throat. It will reduce pain and heal affected area.

Green Tea

Like the vegetables listed above, Japanese green tea contains antioxidants, flavonoids, and substances called indoles, all of which stimulate the body's production of enzymes that block tumor formation.

Milk Thistle

One of the most revered liver cleansers and promoters of liver function in the plant kingdom, milk thistle is used by herbalists to promote the regeneration of the liver. The liver can lose up to three-quarters of its functional capacity and regenerate itself entirely. Milk thistle promotes that regeneration and restoration of the liver.

Mint

Mint is a mild immune booster. Dr. James Duke reports that mint increases the number of phagocyte cells, which are capable of destroying pathogens, bacteria, and cancer cells.

Miso

Miso soup is highly alkaline and supportive of stomach, spleen, and intestinal function, according to Oriental medicine. It promotes healthy digestion and, according to recent research, blocks tumors from forming or advancing.

Oil of Cloves

Brush oil of cloves onto tooth and gum to reduce and eliminate toothache pain. Pain is relieved within a few minutes.

Sage

Used to treat skin problems, especially pimples and acne, sage is antiseptic, anti-inflammatory, and kills bacteria. Usually found as an ingredient in an herbal skin cream or salve.

Salt Water

Use one teaspoon of salt in a cup of hot water to treat sore throats and mouth sores. Gargle and rinse.

Saw Palmetto

One of the most well-studied herbs now available, saw palmetto has been shown to significantly reduce or eliminate symptoms of swollen prostate gland. In tests that compared saw palmetto to existing drugs, saw palmetto was at least as effective as the drugs and caused no ill side effects. In many cases it was more effective. Available in both pills and tinctures in most natural foods and health food stores. Also available now in many pharmacies.

Shiitake Mushrooms

Studies at the U.S. National Cancer Institute and the Japanese National Cancer Institute have established the shiitake mushroom as an immune booster, a cancer fighter, and a powerful cholesterol-lowering herb. Shiitake has antiviral and antibacterial properties. It also causes the immune system to mount a stronger attack against an invading antigen or a tumor. Both animal and human studies have shown that shiitake substantially lowers blood cholesterol. Some research suggests that the cholesterol-lowering effect of shiitake extract—the concentrated form of the herb—may be as much as twenty-five percent when used over a couple of weeks.

Use shiitake mushrooms—either fresh or dried—in soup, stews, and as part of vegetable medleys.

Tea Tree Oil

Tea Tree Oil—a broad spectrum fungicide and antiseptic—is highly effective against a wide variety of skin problems, including acne. The oil is derived from the leaves of the *Melaleuca alternifolia,* a tree that grows in New South Wales, Australia. It is also used to treat bruises and to prevent infection in wounds. For children or those with sensitive skin, Tea Tree Oil can be diluted with water or vegetable oil.

Umeboshi (Plums or Paste)

Used to treat all types of stomach problems, especially simple indigestion, *umeboshi* alkalizes the stomach instantly; calms and soothes. Eat ½ to 1 pickled plum; or eat ⅓ to ½ tsp. of *umeboshi* paste when stomach is distressed. You can also make a tea by combining *kukicha* tea, *umeboshi* paste or plum (same quantities), and two drops of tamari. The tea alkalizes and soothes the stomach.

Witch Hazel

Used to treat many types of skin irritations, rashes, and hemorrhoids, witch hazel is highly astringent. It shrinks vessels and hemorrhoids. Apply frequently during the day or night.

Yarrow

Yarrow is used to treat all types of skin problems, including pimples, acne, infections, itching, rashes, and other skin irritations. It heals and acts as a styptic, a substance that reduces blood flow and inflammation to the area. Usually found as part of an herbal salve that includes other medicinal herbs, such as goldenseal, chamomile, and sage.

Yellowdock

Used traditionally to promote liver cleansing and the health of the colon, yellowdock is a mild laxative. Yellowdock is used primarily to help support and restore liver function and improve iron metabolism of blood. Often used for people suffering from anemia. Take 10 to 30 drops in a tincture, three to five days per week, for two weeks.

Lifestyle Considerations

- Walk daily, weather permitting.

- Get plenty of aerobic exercise, such as bicycling, tennis, swimming, hiking, and running.

- Place plenty of plants throughout the house.

- Sing a happy song every day.

- Chew every mouthful of food thirty-five to fifty times.

- Get regular acupressure, shiatsu, or other forms of body-work therapy.

- Wear only cotton undergarments.

- Avoid eating at least three hours before bed.

Menu Suggestions

Here are menu suggestions that I use in my daily diet. In general, each day, I have a whole-grain food with my breakfast, lunch, and dinner. I also eat noodles, either in broth or with some type of sauce. I eat at least four servings of vegetables daily; at least one serving of beans or bean products; small but regular amounts of fruit and fish; and a wide assortment of condiments. Of course, I use various combinations of these on a regular basis and encourage you to experiment with your own ideas.

Keep in mind that larger quantities of food can be cooked on weekends, at night, or whenever there is enough time to produce a large pot of grain (such as brown rice or barley), a bean, a grain or vegetable stew, and soup. These foods can be reheated throughout the week. In addition, healthful "fast foods" can be prepared in minutes. There are numerous cookbooks with recipes for quick meals that can be prepared in under thirty minutes. These include noodle dishes, steamed or sautéed vegetables (requires less than seven minutes), tofu and tempeh as bean dishes, precooked beans that can be purchased in jars and reheated; quick-cooking grains, such as bulgur, couscous, and buckwheat; and a wide assortment of prepackaged foods that can be made in minutes.

Menu Plan

BREAKFAST

- Miso soup: with *wakame* seaweed and one of a variety of other vegetables, including onions, carrots, and scallions.

- Oatmeal, mixed with raisins, rice syrup (if desired sweet), bulgur wheat, millet, natto, or miso.

- Brown rice, made with more water than the dinner rice (or dinner rice can be reheated with more water to make it wetter and looser for the morning meal).

- Brown rice, mixed with millet, oats, or bulgur wheat.

Note: If your health is good, raisins can be added to the oatmeal to make it sweeter. A small amount, less than a tea-

spoon, of yinnie *rice syrup can be added to the grain on oc-casion, as well.*

LUNCH

- A whole grain: brown rice, millet, barley, or corn (see grains section).

- A green vegetable: Collards, kale, mustard greens, turnip greens, and broccoli are among the best.

- A root or squash or some other vegetable: can include carrots, daikon, or some other vegetable named in veg-etable section.

- A piece of fresh fruit, preferably in season.

DINNER

- A whole grain: Brown rice can be eaten regularly. Other grains should be used, as well. Rice can also be mixed with some beans, including *aduki* beans and lentils. (See grain section for suggestions and cooking instructions.)

- A leafy green: collards, kale, mustard greens, turnip greens, or some other green vegetable.

- A root or squash: See root and squash section. A root and a squash can be eaten at the same meal and can be cooked together, as with acorn squash and carrots. A yellow vegetable, either a squash or carrot, should be eaten four to seven times per week.

- A bean: See bean section for suggestions.

- Fish: Usually small servings are best (3 oz. per serving). It is preferable to make whole grain the center or staple of the diet. For people who are just beginning macrobiotics and are in the habit of eating meat daily, fish can be used as a transition from animal food to grain. Whitefish, haddock, cod, and flounder are preferred because they are lower in fat than most redfish.

DESSERT

- See dessert section for suggestions.

Many can experience a significant improvement in health by adopting these dietary recommendations. Diet is one of the most powerful tools for healing. It is not the only tool, however. We must get regular exercise and learn coping skills to handle our fears. Many feel their lives are incomplete without some sense of union or connection with their own concept of the divine. Once you have adopted a healing diet, I urge you to take the next step in your healing process by adopting an exercise program, which is the subject of our next chapter.

CHAPTER 12

Exercise for Health

A very important component of my own healing was exercise. I believe it's essential for everyone who wants to improve his or her health. I began as soon as possible after my diagnosis, even though light walking was all I could do.

You do not have to do much exercise in order to benefit from it. Nor do you have to adopt any heart-pounding regimen. All you need to do is thirty to forty minutes of walking, four or five times per week. A thirty-minute walk, with arms swinging, can strengthen your muscles, respiration, heart, and circulatory system. Like most forms of exercise, especially those that require you to breathe more rapidly, walking also significantly reduces stress.

Walking, like all aerobic exercise, increases the flow of oxygen to your cells and organs, including your heart and brain. It increases the efficiency of your heart—meaning the heart pumps more blood per beat—and it slows your overall heart rate, which means your heart doesn't have to work as hard all day long.

Exercise also changes the kind of cholesterol in your blood by increasing your HDL levels. HDL, or high density lipoproteins, reduces your risk of heart attack and stroke and consequently is often referred to as the "good" cholesterol. Exercise also promotes better blood flow within your system by reducing the stickiness between blood platelets. This prevents the blood from sludging and getting blocked in the tiny capillaries that bring blood and oxygen to most of your tissues throughout your body.

Exercise also helps to dissolve blood clots, the primary cause of heart attacks and strokes. For these and other reasons, people who exercise tend to have lower heart disease, and other major illnesses, research has shown.

As we all know, exercise burns calories. But did you know that it also helps lower your weight by forcing your body to burn fat as part of its fuel mix long after you have stopped exercising? A thirty to forty-minute bout of exercise will cause you to burn more fat throughout most of the day.

Regular exercise makes your bones stronger and thicker and less likely to fracture. Therefore, exercise is a major factor in the prevention of osteoporosis.

Studies have shown that people who exercise are better able to maintain healthy diets than those who do not exercise. Research has also shown that regular exercise is also associated with lower rates of cancer.

Good for the Body and Mind

Exercise can have a dramatic and positive effect on your mental well-being. As many already know, exercise promotes the secretion of endorphins, which create the so-called "natural high" experienced by virtually anyone who exercises regularly. Endorphins, produced after about twenty minutes of brisk walking, or the equivalent of some other form of aerobic activity, have been shown to act as an antidote to depression and anxiety.

The medical journal *Postgraduate Medicine* reported a

study in their July 1990 issue in which people who had suffered from chronic depression and ongoing stress, including anxiety and emotional disturbances, had fewer bouts of all of these disorders after they began exercising. The people in the study were better able to ward off negative feelings and thoughts after they began a regular exercise routine, the researchers found. The participants felt significantly healthier, more positive, optimistic, and emotionally brighter after they began exercising.

Regular exercise has a unique capacity to strengthen the will and to make us realize that we have the power to change our lives for the better.

The Greatest Exercise of All

For most people, walking is by far the simplest and easiest form of exercise to sustain. We are natural walkers. Few other forms of exercise give us so much pleasure, relaxation, and relief from stress and negative emotions. This is especially true when we walk in a beautiful, natural environment. A walk in a beautiful park, across a serene woods, or along a beach, can have an overpowering effect on us. It takes over our mood and alchemically transforms us from within.

Whenever you walk, do not strain or stress yourself beyond your capacity. When you feel a need to rest, slow down, or stop and catch your breath. Sit for a time and allow your body to recover. For those who are not used to exercising, strolling is the best form of exercise.

A good test to see if you are overexerting yourself is to see if you can talk while walking. If you are short of breath or winded, you will not be able to talk, but if you can talk and walk, you are not overexerting yourself.

Walk: It Could Save Your Life

The November 1988 *Journal of the American Medical Association* reported a study that examined the effects of exercise on mortality rates. The study, done by the Institute for Aerobic Research in Dallas, Texas, followed 13,344 men and women for eight years. The participants were divided into five groups, based on the amount of exercise they did each week. One group did no exercise at all; a second group walked four to six times per week; the next two groups participated to varying degrees in athletics or fitness programs; the fifth group was made up of marathoners or high-intensity athletes.

All the participants were tested on treadmills to determine their fitness levels and categorized accordingly in one of the five groups. For eight years scientists followed the five groups and determined which group had the highest mortality rates.

As expected, the scientists found that the death rate was highest among those who were least fit, the sedentary group. What the scientists didn't expect was that the greatest difference in mortality existed between those who were sedentary and those who simply walked four to six times per week. They found that the sedentary group had three times more deaths than the walking group had. After the enormous difference in mortality between these two groups, the differences in the next three groups—all of whom were athletes or intense exercisers—were relatively small.

"Even modest amounts of exercise can substantially reduce a person's chances of dying" of heart disease, cancer, and other illnesses, reported the November 3, 1989, *New York Times.* "This is a hopeful message, an important message for the American people to understand," Dr. Carl Caspersen, of the Federal Centers for Disease Control, told *The New York Times.* "You don't have to be a marathoner. In fact, you get much more benefit out of being just a bit more active. For example, going from being sedentary to walking briskly for a half hour several days a week can drop your risk dramatically."

Weight Training

Researchers at the Massachusetts Institute of Technology have found that people well into their nineties benefit from resistance or weight training. Weight training builds bone and makes muscles stronger and bigger. With increased muscle mass and strength, people are less likely to fall, and if they do, they are less likely to break a bone. Muscle is also active tissue; it breaks down and burns fat, even while it is resting. Weight training increases HDL levels, strengthens the heart, increases the metabolic rate, boosts stamina and strength. With increased strength comes dramatically increased confidence and self-esteem. I highly recommend it.

If you are new to weight training, do what I did: work with the bar alone, or five-pound weights that can be held in your hand. Talk to someone who can guide you effectively in your resistance training. Virtually all fitness clubs have a weight-training expert on hand to lead you through an array of exercises that will benefit every muscle and bone in your body.

See Your Doctor Before You Stress Your Heart

A little preventive medicine never hurt. If you are out of shape, have high blood pressure, smoke cigarettes, have a history of heart disease, take medication, or are under medical supervision for any condition, see your doctor before you begin an exercise program.

Do not engage in competitive sports, at least initially. Competition makes us forget ourselves and push harder than wisdom might recommend. Get yourself in good condition before you take on the neighbor in a game of tennis or basketball.

There's a Whole World of Healthy Activity Out There

There are so many forms of exercise out there that all of us can find an activity that we enjoy, thereby improving our health and sustaining it. Here are some guidelines to help you find that pastime that can change your life for the better, and perhaps lengthen it, too.

1. The first rule: Have fun! Most of us are not out there to become Olympic athletes. We're engaging in an exercise-activity to enjoy ourselves and improve our health. If it isn't fun, it cannot be sustained, so you're wasting your time. Pick up that game you have always wanted to start. Begin a martial art, such as Tai Chi Chuan. Dance. Walk. Lift a few weights a couple of times per week. Make it fun and it will change your life.
2. Use the right equipment—comfortable and supportive shoes, light and loose clothing, and a place to exercise that is safe and enriching to you.
3. If possible, walk with a friend. Walking with a friend will keep both of you on track. When you walk with someone else, you're getting the cheapest form of therapy there is. Walking alone relieves physical, mental, and emotional stress. The company of someone you enjoy, who shares his or her thoughts, is an added blessing.
4. Dance! There are few things more aerobic and joyful. Start slowly and gradually increase the level of intensity as your conditioning improves. Do not tax yourself excessively, especially in the beginning.

5. Join a club. There are fitness clubs, tennis and racquetball clubs, nature walking and hiking clubs, and clubs for seniors. Local recreation organizations sponsor walking and hiking trips. YMCAs offer everything from basketball and volleyball to swimming and water aerobics. There are endless classes for yoga, aerobic dance, stretching, and other forms of exercise. These clubs and classes are usually inexpensive and are great ways to meet people. If possible, join a fitness, racquetball, tennis, or golf club and take lessons. One of the great joys of sport is that your skills can improve, which is part of the ongoing enjoyment of the game.

6. Riding a bike is still one of the most enjoyable forms of exercise you will ever experience. Highly aerobic, bicycling can be a very demanding form of exercise. People who are out of shape should start out on flat surfaces and ride only for short distances until they build their conditioning and endurance. It's important to get your bicycle in order, as well. A bike shop can tune your bike and make it far more pleasant to ride. Bicycling is addictive; once you get into the habit, you won't want to stop.

7. Purchase a treadmill or a stationary bike. Treadmills and stationary bicycles allow you to exercise right in your own home. You can watch television, listen to music, listen to self-help tapes, or meditate as you walk or pedal. Many treadmills and stationary bicycles today provide all kinds of information, including miles traveled and calories burned. You can change the pitch on a treadmill to increase or decrease the intensity of the exercise. Treadmills also allow you to run without resistance. (The conveyor actually moves your leg back, rather than your having to push yourself forward.) Both treadmills and stationary bicycles provide great workouts, and many people who use them maintain that they wouldn't exercise at all were it not for

the availability of their machine right in their own home.

8. Before you begin, warm up. It only takes ten minutes to do so, but it will protect your body from injury and make it easier for you to walk or exercise longer.

9. Whether you're playing tennis, basketball, or just walking, start out slowly, at a leisurely pace, and increase your effort as your muscles stretch and adjust to the exercise. Don't push yourself excessively. It will only increase the likelihood of injury. Rest whenever you feel the need.

10. After you finish, cool down. Walk slowly, stretch for ten minutes, and then walk some more to allow your muscles to relax and slowly cool down. Abrupt finishes after exercise can cause you to cramp or cause muscles to go into spasm.

When it comes to any exercise, keep the first rule upper most in your mind: Have fun! It's the best guide to any exercise activity you can do.

CHAPTER 13

Facing the Demons Within: Handling Stress

I began my own recovery process by adopting a healing diet and re-entering therapy. I also exercised, did yoga, got massages, read inspirational books, meditated, and prayed daily. This routine gave me a degree of inner peace, though I must admit that fear was always close to my consciousness, if not occupying center stage. Over time, however, the degree of stress and fear I experienced diminished considerably. I began to develop a growing faith.

That is the essence of what I was looking for—what most of us are looking for, I daresay. Faith is an antidote to fear.

When I say faith, I mean a conviction that the universe is essentially benevolent and supportive of my life—that life, in the largest sense, is leading me toward the resolution of my problems. With faith, we feel that circumstances are leading us toward the realization of our most cherished dreams and therefore our greatest happiness. Faith assures us that this is true, even when all that we are dealing with seems like a problem itself.

Most of us live by the opposite conviction: Everything around us is falling apart, and life is heading toward some unknown and as yet undefined disaster. Even when disaster doesn't strike, that belief is highly destructive and incredibly stress-provoking. As Albert Einstein said, all of us must answer the same question: Is the universe a friendly place? If your answer is no, then your're in for a rough ride. Given the power of external events to control our lives, and given the awesome capacity for the unexpected event to suddenly turn our lives into chaos, the thought of an unfriendly universe is terrifying, to say the least. It is essentially a living hell. Interestingly, when looked at carefully, our experience of hell may not be so much because our external circumstances are difficult, but because our inner lives are in turmoil. As Krishnamurti used to say, most of us, most of the time, are perfectly safe. Right now, for example, you may be sitting in your home reading this book and be living—at least in this particular moment—in the safest circumstances possible. It is our negative expectations about the future that cause us fear or stress.

My point is that expectations, negative or positive, very often determine our inner worlds and, for that matter, the degree of stress we experience. Science has demonstrated this to be true. Once we have been subjected to a powerful, stressful experience—such as sickness or chemotherapy treatments—we can become weakened by the mere thought of those treatments. Like the bell in Pavlov's experiments, the thought of such events triggers a physical and immune-depressing reaction within the body. Studies have shown that cancer patients who have undergone chemotherapy treatments tend to suffer nausea or vomiting from the mere anticipation of the next round of chemotherapy drugs. Other research has shown that that same anticipation also weakens immune response. Thus, the mere anticipation of a negative event can lower our resistance to disease and our ability to fight it off.

You do not have to have cancer or some other serious illness to experience stress. Researchers have consistently shown that exams lower the immune response of college students. The number and effectiveness of several types of important immune cells is weakened when the system is subjected to prolonged stress. Other research has shown that common tasks, such as job interviews, also weaken immune response.

Most of us experience it every day of our lives. Those of us who are chronically distressed are continually depressing our immune systems, and thus increasing our chances of becoming ill.

Stress weakens immune response and thereby raises the likelihood that you will become infected with a virus or bacteria, including the common cold. Chronic stress also makes you more vulnerable to contracting a degenerative disease, such as heart disease, high blood pressure, cancer, asthma, diabetes, and inflammatory bowel disease. Growing numbers of researchers and doctors believe that stress plays a role in the onset of multiple sclerosis, rheumatoid arthritis, and other autoimmune diseases, though these links have yet to be proven.

A variety of immune functions are influenced by stress. Recently a team of researchers reviewed thirty-eight well-controlled studies that examined the effects of stress on the immune system and concluded that the evidence demonstrates that the immune systems of people under stress is clearly weaker.

The studies show that people who are subjected to stress have weaker immune responses than those who are not subjected to stress. Scientists have consistently shown that the number of natural killer (NK) cells decrease. These cells play a major role in the body's ability to fight off cancer, as well as viruses and bacteria.

Messenger chemicals that make communication within the immune system possible also decrease as a result of stress. This makes the overall immune response weaker and more confused.

Chronic stress has been shown to make viruses, such as

herpes and HIV, stronger and more active. At the same time, stress weakens the immune system, which increases the likelihood that such viruses can gain sway over the body.

The immune system is directed by a group of immune cells called CD4 cells. These cells, often referred to as the "generals of the immune system," organize the immune system's response to a disease-causing agent, such as a bacteria, virus, or cancer cell. When the disease has been defeated, CD8 cells arise to turn off the immune system, lest it begin attacking and destroying the body, as well. A number of studies have shown that stress lowers the number of CD4 and elevates the number of CD8 cells, meaning that it weakens the generals and increases the cells whose job it is to turn off the system.

Stress can have a profound effect on hormones. Hormones produced under stress can promote cardiovascular disease, immune dysfunction, anxiety, excitation, rapid heart beat, and respiration. These hormones can contribute to aging, depression, and certain autoimmune diseases, such as asthma and arthritis.

Mind Boosters to Boost Your Immune System

For all of these reasons, all of us, no matter what our current health status may be, need some antidote to stress. We need to cultivate behaviors that strengthen our faith. Fortunately, there are many powerful tools that not only reduce stress, but also strengthen the immune system in the process.

Daily meditation and relaxation exercises, such as the progressive releasing of tension in the muscles, cause CD4 cells to increase in number, researchers at the University of Miami Medical School have found. Scientists there examined the effects of stress and progressive relaxation on men with HIV, an illness that normally decreases the number of CD4 cells. Researchers found that daily meditation and progressive relaxation exercises increased the number of CD4 cells, and thereby strengthened the immune system dramatically. When the scientists followed up on the men a year later, they found that those who continued to meditate or do the relaxation exercises were less likely to have progressed to full-blown AIDS.

One study found that medical students who practiced daily relaxation routines experienced an increase in the number of natural killer and CD4 cells.

According to Ellen Langer, a psychologist at Harvard University, transcendental meditation—a practice in which a single word or phrase is repeated silently over and over again—creates deep states of relaxation and may increase longevity. Langer followed people living in nursing homes to see what effect, if any, TM would have on longevity. After three years, Langer found that all the members of a group that practiced TM were still alive, while only thirty-eight percent of those who did not practice TM were alive.

Herbert Benson, M.D., associate professor of medicine at Harvard Medical School, has found that ten to twenty minutes of meditation per day lowers blood pressure, slows heart rate, relaxes muscles, and creates a more balanced hormonal condition. All of these traits can contribute to a stronger immune response.

The following techniques, when practiced regularly, can boost your immune system and protect you against disease. In addition to these, I encourage you to develop your own practices that make you feel relaxed and peaceful and help you develop faith. Consider, as well, attending some kind of traditional service that you feel drawn to. Many churches, synagogues, and mosques are permeated with a spirit that instantly transforms our internal condition the moment we walk into them. Walk into a place of worship, even when there is no service going on, and meditate or pray for a short while and notice the effects such a place has on you.

Practicing these techniques in nature, such as in the forest, by a river, or at the ocean, can also have a very powerful and transformational effect on us. I encourage you to experiment with all of these possibilities, as well as with many different techniques until you find what works for you.

The Breath: A Vehicle to Inner Peace

One of the simplest and most powerful tools for relaxation and meditation is simply watching and concentrating on your breath. You can do this at any moment of the day. When you sit down at your desk or get into your car, stop everything for a moment and exhale. Drop your shoulders and notice how much tension you can release simply by letting go of the out breath and relaxing your shoulder muscles. The experience can be powerful. It's as if you reenter your body suddenly and are present in the here and now.

You can observe your breath as a means of meditation and deep relaxation.

Begin by sitting on a comfortable seat, or a pillow, or a soft part of the earth, in a place that will help you relax and will prevent you from being distracted. Inhale deeply and allow a long, relaxing exhale. Watch yourself inhale and exhale rhythmically. Feel the relaxation settle on you as you watch your breath.

Observe any thoughts that may come to mind. As best you can, avoid engaging the thoughts that arise. Instead, simply witness each thought as it arises and leaves your consciousness. Each thought is a passing cloud. It appears and softly drifts away.

As you do this exercise, you will eventually notice various emotions begin to emerge, very often from the lower part of your body or your heart area. Feel the feeling and then let it go. Make no judgments about any particular memory or thought that comes into your mind. Let each feeling, memory, or thought emerge and then dissolve away. Do not engage it; do not invest any of your life energy into anything.

You are only sitting and watching your breath. You are observing and releasing.

When you find yourself entering into an emotion or thought, come back to your breath. Breathe deeply; exhale. Allow the deep relaxation to release every bit of tension in your body.

Author and medical pioneer Dean Ornish, M.D., director of the Preventive Medicine Research Institute in Sausalito, California, says that "deep breathing is one of the simplest, yet most effective stress-management techniques there is." Ornish, whose vegetarian diet is very similar to the macrobiotic program I used to treat my cancer, recommends deep breathing and yoga as fundamental to a healing program.

The Power of a Mantra

Concentrate on and repeat a mantra, a single word or phrase, slowly and rhythmically. Let it crowd out all other thoughts and feelings until it brings you into a deep state of relaxation and peace. Chanting the word or phrase can help you with concentration. Among the words many people use are God, Jesus, Mother Mary, om, shalom (the Hebrew word for peace), *Nam Myo Ho Renge Kyo* (a popular Buddhist chant thought to be very empowering), and the names of common spiritual and religious figures.

Your Mind's Peaceful Place

Go to a place in your home or some other setting where you will not be disturbed. Sit on a comfortable chair, or on some pillows on the floor, or a soft place on the earth, and breathe deeply. Watch your breath for a time until you are fully relaxed. Now, focus for as long as you can on a specific place—either a place you know, or somewhere in your imagination—that conveys relaxation, peace, and tranquillity. Enjoy this place. Walk around in your mind. Notice all its details and the feelings that arise in you as you examine this place.

Many people who do this exercise encounter someone special in this place—a long-lost relative, a spiritual guide, or a religious figure. If that is the case for you, talk to this person. Convey your fears and ask for help. Surrender into the embrace of this loving figure.

Biofeedback

Biofeedback is a powerful tool for releasing tension and achieving deep states of relaxation. Psychotherapists, health centers, colleges, and universities in your community offer biofeedback training. Like the meditation techniques I have described, biofeedback uses visualization to induce relaxation. In the case of biofeedback, certain technological devices are used to help you observe and learn to control your body temperature, perspiration, heart rate, and other physical symptoms. In time you can learn how to use your mind to control how your body responds to various types of situations, especially those that cause you stress.

Biofeedback is an effective treatment for a wide array of illnesses, including angina, anxiety, asthma, intestinal disorders, chronic pain, epilepsy, headaches and migraines, high blood pressure, high cholesterol, insomnia, learning disabilities, muscle spasm, phobias, rapid heart rate, TMJ (temporomandibular joint dysfunction), and urinary problems.

Support Groups

Studies have shown that women who are coping with breast cancer and join a support group live up to two years longer, on average, than those who avoid such groups. Other research has demonstrated that support groups strengthen immune response. One of the essential parts of any healing program is support from others. Do not attempt to heal yourself on your own. No one can do this work by himself. We need the love, encouragement, perspective, experience, talent, and insight of others in order to find our way back to health. Illnesses of all types flourish when we are isolated.

Support groups can be found in the Yellow Pages, through cancer hotlines, Twelve Step programs (such as Alcoholics Anonymous and Adult Children of Alcoholics), local churches, synagogues, and other religious organizations.

The Healing Touch

One of the most essential parts of my own healing program was to have an experienced, knowledgeable body-work practitioner work on me on a weekly basis. In most cases these people are trained professionals with a deep commitment to health and healing. There are endless numbers of body-work therapies. Among the most common are acupressure, Alexander technique, dance movement therapies, energy healing, Feldenkrais method, Hellerwork, *Jin Shin Jyutsu*, kinesiology, neuromuscular therapy, *Ohashiatsu*, physical and occupational therapies, polarity therapy, reflexology, Reiki, Rolfing, The Rubenfeld Synergy, shiatsu, Swedish massage, therapeutic touch, and Trager.

Healing touch is especially powerful for those who are eating well, meditating, and working to better understand and experience their bodies. But even for those who are on the go and don't want to think about their health, body work can be a powerful tool for relaxation, elimination of stress and tension, and a wonderful way to restore balance in your life.

Funny Movies, Theater, and Stand-up

Laughter strengthens the immune system, relaxes muscles, and changes biochemistry for the better. Laughter triggers the production of endorphins, the opiatelike chemicals that provide feelings of well-being and the so-called natural high. It can also lower blood pressure.

Research at the University of California at Santa Barbara found that laughter was just as effective at reducing stress as biofeedback training. Scientists are finding that even changing your facial expression from a frown to a smile directly alters mood for the better. Researchers at Clark University at Worcester, Massachusetts, found that simply having people adopt the facial expression of a particular mood actually created that mood in the people themselves. Expressions of fear brought on feelings of fear and stress.

Warm Baths for Relaxation

Warm water relaxes muscles, improves circulation, and slightly warms the brain, which scientists say is calming to the entire system. The water temperature should not exceed 102° F. Excess heat can be shocking to the system, causing muscles to contract while increasing circulation—an unhealthy combination. Soak in the tub for no more than fifteen minutes. (Those with diabetes should avoid hot baths entirely.) Pour sea salt or mineral salts in the water to keep the water from draining minerals from your body. Bath salts are available in most natural-foods stores. Also add aromatherapy products from time to time to enhance relaxation and promote healing.

The following is a sample of meditations and guided imagery exercises that you can use.

Guided Imagery Exercise No. 1

Relaxation Exercise

- Sit in a comfortable chair, on a pillow, or on soft ground. Take off your shoes.

- Observe your breathing and allow it to come into a natural, relaxed rhythm.

- Bring your attention to the muscles in your face. Allow them to relax. Let the tension in your face melt away.

- Next, allow the muscles in your neck and shoulders to relax. Feel your shoulders drop into their natural place. Notice how dropping your shoulders affects your breath. Feel the tension drain from your entire upper body.

- Allow your hands and arms to relax in your lap. Visualize the tension draining from your hands and arms.

- Turn your attention to your chest and stomach area. Breathe deeply into your stomach. Observe in your mind's eye the rise and fall of your stomach. Feel your chest muscles relax. Observe your breath. Feel your stomach muscles relax. Again, observe your breath. Feel your center of gravity fall into the lower part of your abdomen.

- Feel any tension that may be in your legs and feet. Allow your legs to relax. Let the tension drain from your thighs, calves, ankles, and feet. Watch it seep from the bottoms of your feet and into the earth.

- Feel your body as an integrated whole, feel its unity and how deeply relaxed you are right now.

- In your imagination, take yourself to a favorite place in nature—a forest, near a river, the ocean, or the desert. Observe this place in detail. Feel the earth at your feet, the air on your skin, and every natural detail in your immediate environment.

- Hold the image of this place as long as you can in your mind and enjoy being in this place. You have all the

time in the world. There are no pressing matters to at-
tend to. There's nothing more important right now
than simply being in this place. Allow this place, with
all its beauty and mystery, to feed you life-supportive
energy. Be here until your spirit tells you it's time to go.

Guided Imagery Exercise No. 2

The Light Meditation

- Perform the Relaxation Exercise previously described.

- "See" a small beam of life emerge from your heart area.

- Notice that this light is very powerful and growing.
  Realize that it is connected to an infinite source of
  healing energy.

- Observe that this beam of light is alive. It is a kind of
  light-filled, viscous elixir that is filling your heart and
  chest area.

- Observe that it is radiating out from your chest,
  spreading a powerful healing energy throughout your
  chest area. It is filling your heart and every cell with
  joy, love, and limitless energy.

- Watch this powerful light-energy expand upward
  through your neck and into your head so that it completely fills the upper part of your body with light, joy,
  and healing energy.

- In the same way, watch the light come down into your
  arms and hands, permeating every cell with this healing energy.

- Watch it move down from your chest like a flowing river into your lower abdomen, sex organs, legs, and feet. Observe how it unifies, strengthens, and restores every cell that it imbues.

- See how weakened and darkened cells become light-filled, vital, and fully alive again.

- Watch this light as it flows through your blood. See it embracing and infusing every cell in your blood stream, including your oxygen-carrying red blood cells and the white cells of your immune system. Picture each cell becoming clothed in light, energy, and healing power.

- Picture the light cells transforming every diseased cell into yet another version of the light-filled, vital, and fully alive cells. Every cell in your body is being transformed into light, energy, and love.

- Observe how your entire body is now engulfed in light.

- Picture a large but distinct source of light just above your head. You are suddenly aware of this light-filled source as a living entity that is sending you an infinite supply of love and healing energy. The love is completely unconditional. There are no judgments, only love and warmth and happiness.

- Imagine this source of light sending its healing energy pouring into your being so that the light that filled your body is now ten times brighter and now a hundred times brighter.

- Bathe in the warmth of this energy. It is love.

- Continue the meditation until your spirit tells you it's time to relax.

- Breathe deeply and release all emotion that may have come up during the meditation.

Illness, I came to realize, is a kind of separation from myself. I thought of my disease as another life-form that was living inside me. But unlike a child, this life-form was attempting to destroy me. The illness was separate and antagonistic.

Healing is unifying and bringing our disparate parts back into the light of love and acceptance. All healing, therefore, flows from love. Part of the healing process is to become aware of those memories and characteristics in ourselves that we deny, reject, and may even hate. These separated aspects of ourselves live in darkness and in isolation, there they breed disease and ultimately lead to our demise.

There is nothing inside of us that cannot be understood and welcomed back into consciousness and love. This is the most basic and essential work of healing. For in the end, all of us come to realize that love is really the healer.

CHAPTER 14

Spiritual Healing

My book is a story of a spiritual transformation. All the details of this transformation, or as many as I understand and am able to relate, are provided throughout my story. What I urge people to do first, is to find a practice that meets their spiritual needs. Second, do all they can to restore balance in their lives. The tools that I offer in this section are ways to do exactly that.

Healing oneself begins as a process of peeling away one layer at a time, discovering how we have physically and mentally imprisoned ourselves. The effect, however, of liberating yourself from those self-imposed limits is not to increase your sense of controlling your destiny. My "terminal" cancer sentence caused me to realize how little control I had over my destiny. The control I had so carefully exercised over my life turned out to be killing me! Losing the arrogance of "being in control" and searching for the universal connection with all life that is within each of us was perhaps my hardest lesson.

The greatest irony I experienced in ridding myself of cancer was embracing the necessity of giving up control of my life and health, giving it up not to doctors but to an infinite force. The irony was in the fact that all the new ways of eating, exercising, and even counseling seemed to be directed at getting a new control of my life. But soon after I was diagnosed as "terminal," I realized that all the efforts at controlling my life had produced the dangerous situation I was in. I reexamined my previously superficial commitment to my Catholic faith and found it wanting. This time I approached God from a position of complete acceptance and openness. I accepted my mortality and only asked God to direct my life, whatever that course might be.

It was in this openness that I realized balance was the key to spiritual harmony.

Unfortunately, the term "balance" has been thrown around so much in healing today that it may have lost its meaning for many of us. How many of us really make choices according to any concept of balance? Yet, there are several ways of using balance to understand ourselves and the amount of stress in our lives. According to Chinese healers, one way of seeking balance is to ask ourselves whether we expend more energy than we gather. Do we engage in activities that demand more physical, emotional, and intellectual investment than they give back as rewards? Do we engage in activities that leave us feeling empty and exhausted at the end of the day?

Another way to seek balance is to understand how we use our time. Does our work completely eclipse all opportunities to play, or to experience intimacy with ourselves and others?

Redford Williams, M.D., director of Behavioral Research at Duke University Medical School, found that those who suffer a heart attack and have no spouse or close personal friend are more apt to have a fatal heart attack within five years of the original event than those whose hearts are equally injured but are married or have intimate relationships. "What we found was that those patients with neither a spouse nor a friend were three times more likely to die than those involved in a caring relationship," said Dr. Williams.

Other research has consistently supported these findings. Women with breast cancer who participate in a support group live longer than those who try to deal with the disease alone. Scientists are discovering that not only are the recommendations of traditional healers effective, but so, too, are the guidelines for living offered by spiritual traditions. After reviewing the evidence linking meditation and intimacy to longer life, Dr. Williams said, "It seems evident that the core teachings of most of our religions have been right all along."

Try the following exercise to understand your imbalances: Draw a circle and divide it into segments that represent the amount of time you devote to five key areas of your life:

1. The time you devote to your work and career.
2. The time and energy you devote to your intimate relationships, such as your lover and/or immediate family members, such as children.
3. The time and attention you devote to your friendships.
4. The time devoted to play.
5. The time you have for yourself to be alone, to do whatever you enjoy doing for yourself, and to reconnect with yourself and your life, allowing your own needs to surface.

After drawing the circle with its five segments, recognize where your life is imbalanced. Take each segment of your life that is currently neglected and commit to giving that segment an hour to two hours in a single day during the week ahead. It's common, for example, to devote more time and energy to career than to any other pastime. Loved ones and friends may feel neglected. But even more fundamentally, those who devote an excessive amount of their lives to their career neglect themselves in very basic ways. There's little or no time to play, contemplate one's life, dream, conjure up new and creative ideas, be inspired, or simply *be*—that is, to be intimate with oneself.

Make it a goal for one week to redistribute four hours from the dominant areas of life to those parts of your life that you feel are neglected.

If four hours cannot be redistributed, then redirect as much time as possible to the parts of life that you miss. Among the recommendations to achieve balance are the following:

- Spend an hour or two doing nothing. And do it intentionally and with commitment. All of us spend some time doing nothing, but typically we are not committed to doing nothing for that half hour or hour. We do it unconsciously, usually without planning or even without directly recognizing that we're taking time to rest. Be deliberate. Take an hour and say, "I'm doing nothing now." Stroke your cat; sit in the afternoon sun; let the inner world bubble up into your consciousness.

- No television for a week, especially if you watch a lot. Not only will it free up time, but it will give you back your sense of self.

- Schedule a breakfast, intimate lunch, or romantic dinner with your lover, if time has been low. Go to bed forty-five minutes earlier to talk, or to allow you to get up earlier to have breakfast with your spouse or lover.

- Go to bed an hour earlier to catch up on sleep.

- Call that person with whom you've wanted to develop a friendship and invite him or her to play tennis, watch a film, have a cup of tea, or a glass of beer. The point is to expand your social life and start to develop one closer relationship.

- Send a little long-distance love. Write a letter to a friend or relative you care about but with whom you've been out of touch. Send your love and support.

- Turn your life or your dream into art. With colored pencils, pens, or paints, draw a picture of your inner world, or an image of how you want your life to develop. What does the next step in your life look like? Do you see yourself breaking free or becoming more relaxed or achieving some great dream? Draw an image that expresses the feeling, or shows that you have already accomplished this goal.

- Reward yourself healthfully. Give yourself a special gift that's meant to pamper you: a massage, a facial, a manicure, a pedicure, a hot tub, an acupuncture treatment, an energy healing, a night of dancing, a night at the theater, the symphony, or a rock concert, or a weekend in the country at a special inn.

- Get a cat or a dog and make a lifelong friend. Not only will this boost your immune system, but it will give you years of love and comfort.

To release yourself from a "terminal illness," you must re-examine your spiritual roots and approach the infinite from a position of surrender and serenity: Surrender to the part you are guided to play in life's drama, and accept serenity in the infinite power of God to direct our lives in a purposeful way.

When I was able to see myself as a unique spiral of energy within a never-ending river of energy called life, I was able to surrender to the changes that entered my life. I was able to embrace a new diet and a new relationship with food. I accepted exercise, yoga, breathing, my church, massage, and counseling as vibrant gifts from God to transform my sense of separateness into a recognition of my oneness with all living beings.

Resource Guide

MACROBIOTICS

Cookbooks about Macrobiotics

Meals that Heal by Lisa Turner. (Healing Arts Press)

The Book of Whole Meals by Annemarie Colbin. (Ballantine)

Introducing Macrobiotic Cooking by Ed and Wendy Esko. (Japan Publications)

Macrobiotic Cooking for Everyone by Ed and Wendy Esko. (Japan Publications)

The Complete Guide to Macrobiotic Cooking by Aveline Kushi. (Japan Publications)

Quick and Natural Cookbook by Aveline Kushi. (Japan Publications)

Macrobiotic Kitchen by Cornelia Aihara. (George Ohsawa Macrobiotic Foundation)

First Macrobiotic Cookbook by Cornelia Aihara. (George Ohsawa Macrobiotic Foundation)

Food and Healing by Annemarie Colbin. (Ballantine)

The Self-Healing Cookbook by Kristina Turner.

The Naturally Healthy Gourmet by Margaret Lawson. (George Ohsawa Macrobiotic Association, Oroville, CA)

Natural Foods Cookbook by Mary Estella. (Japan Publications)

Other Books About Macrobiotics

The Cancer Prevention Diet by Michio Kushi, with Alex Jack. (St. Martin's Press)

The Book of Macrobiotics by Michio Kushi with Alex Jack. (St. Martin's Press)

Acid and Alkaline by Herman Aihara. (George Ohsawa Macrobiotic Foundation)

Learning From Salmon by Herman Aihara. (George Ohsawa Macrobiotic Foundation)

Recalled By Life by Dr. Anthony Sattilaro, with Tom Monte. (Avon Books) Available in libraries.

Living Well Naturally by Dr. Anthony Sattilaro, with Tom Monte. (Houghton Mifflin)

World Medicine: The East–West Guide to Healing Your Body by Tom Monte and the editors of *Natural Health.* (Putnam, 1993)

The Way of Hope: Michio Kushi's Anti-AIDS Program by Tom Monte. (Warner Books, 1989)

The Complete Guide to Natural Healing by Tom Monte and the editors of *Natural Health.* (Putnam-Perigee Press)

Macrobiotic Publications and Publishers

George Ohsawa Macrobiotic Foundation (publishers). 1999 Myers Street, Oroville, CA 95966. Tel: 916-533-7702. Fax: 916-533-7908. Publishers of a wide variety of books and cookbooks on macrobiotics.

One Peaceful World Press. P.O. Box 10, Becket, MA 01223. Tel: 413-623-2322. Publishers of a wide variety of books and cookbooks on macrobiotics.

Macrobiotics Today magazine. George Ohsawa Macrobiotic

Foundation. 1999 Myers Street, Oroville, CA 95966. Tel: 916-533-7702. Fax: 916-533-7908

MacroChef. A magazine dedicated solely to macrobiotic cooking. 243 Dickinson Street, Philadelphia, PA 19147.

Macrobiotic Education and Counseling

The Kushi Institute. P.O. Box 7, Becket, MA 01223. Tel: 1-800-97-KUSHI. Office: 413-623-5741. Fax: 413-623-8827.

Vega Study Center, 1511 Robinson Street, Oroville, CA 95965. Tel: 800-818-VEGA (8342) also: 916-533-7702.

Directories of Macrobiotic Teaching Centers, Teachers, Counselors, Restaurants, Food Stores, and other Resources Worldwide

The International Macrobiotic Directory, by Robert Matson. 1050 40th Street, Oakland, CA. Tel: 510-601-1763. Fax: 510-652-0298.

Macrobiotic Health and Travel Directory. One Peaceful World Press. Tel: 413-623-2322. Fax: 413-623-6042.

Web sites

www.macrobiotics.org. for the Kushi Institute and One Peaceful World.

Macrobiotic Food, Cookware, Supplies, and Books by Mail Order

Kushi Institute Store. 1-800-64-Kushi. Macrobiotic foods, cookware, bodycare products, books, videos, and audiotapes.

Gold Mine Natural Food Co. 1800-475-FOOD (3663). Gold Mine Natural Food Co. 3419 Hancock Street San Diego, CA 92110-4307. Tel: 619-296-8536. Fax: 619-296-9756.

Macro Supplies By Mail. 16 Mt. Lookout Drive, Asheville, NC 288804. Tel: 800-752-2775.

GENERAL INFORMATION CANCER AND CANCER TREATMENTS

Information About Cancer

The National Cancer Institute, public information: 1-800-422-6237
Web sites for the National Cancer Institute:
www.nic.nih.gov

Cancer Support Groups

Telephone the National Cancer Institute for a cancer support group in your area: 1-800-422-6237 or 1-800-227-2345.
The National Cancer Institute's Web site for support groups and other information: Http://cancernet.nci.nih.gov

TRADITIONAL AND ALTERNATIVE MEDICINE RESOURCES

Chinese Medicine

American Association of Oriental Medicine. 433 Front Street, Catasauqua, PA 18032. Toll-free tel: 888-500-7999; 610-266-1433; fax: 610-264-2768.
Web site: Http://www.aaom.org
Provides information on all forms of Oriental medicine, including acupuncture, acupressure, and Chinese herbology; as well as a referral service.

American Academy of Medical Acupuncture. 5820 Wilshire Blvd., Suite 500, Los Angeles, CA 90036. 323-937-5514.
Web site: Http//www.medical acupuncture.org

Naturopathy

National College of Naturopathic Medicine. 049 SW Porter, Portland, OR 97201. Tel: 503-499-4343; fax: 503-499-0027.

American Association of Naturopathic Physicians. 601 Valley Street, Suite 105, Seattle, WA 98109. tel: 206-298-0216; fax: 206-298-0129.

Therapeutic Massage

American Massage Therapy Association. 820 Davis Street, Suite 100, Evanston, IL 60201.

National Locator Service. 847-864-0123.
Web site: Http://www.amtamassage.org

Herbology

Books on Herbology

Planetary Herbology by Michael Tierra, C.A., N.D. (Lotus Press, Sante Fe, NM)
Natural Healing with Herbs by Humbart Santillo, N.D. (Hohm Press, Prescott, AZ)

Comprehensive Guides to Healing and Traditional Medicine

Healing with Whole Foods, Oriental Traditions and Modern Nutrition by Paul Pitchford. (North Atlantic Books, Berkeley, CA)
The Complete Guide to Natural Healing by Tom Monte and the editors of *Natural Health*. (Perigee-Putnam Books, New York)

Books on visualization, meditation, and prayer

Healing Words: The Power of Prayer and the Practice of Medicine by Larry Dossey, M.D. (HarperSanFrancisco, San Francisco, CA)

Psychoimmunity and the Healing Process Jason Serinus, editor. (Celestial Arts, Berkeley, CA)

Science of Breath: A Practical Guide by Swami Rama, Rudolph Ballentine, M.D., Alan Hymes, M.D. (The Himalayan International Institute of Yoga Science and Philosophy, Honesdale, PA)

The Bodymind Workbook: Exploring how the mind and the body work together by Debbie Shapiro. (Element Books, Great Britain)

Ordinary Magic: Everyday Life as a Spiritual Path, edited by John Welwood. (Shambhala, Boston, MA)

On-Line Services

For on-line information, resources, and services concerning all forms of traditional and alternative forms of medicine—including naturopathy, herbology, ayurveda, and macrobiotics, and visualization—and for the purchase of foods, herbs, and supplements log on: www.herbal alternatives. com.